Prentice Hall Health

outline review

Medical Assistant

for the

Prentice Hall Health

outline review
Medical Assistant

for the

Second Edition

Marsha Perkins Hemby, BA, RN, CMA
Department Chairman, Medical Assisting
Pitt Community College
Greenville, North Carolina

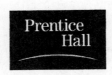

Prentice Hall
Upper Saddle River, New Jersey 07458

Library of Congress Cataloging-in-Publication Data
Hemby, Marsha Perkins.
　Prentice Hall health outline review for the medical
assistant/Marsha Perkins Hemby.—2nd ed.
　　p. cm.
　Previous ed. published as: Medical assisting review.
　Includes bibliographical references and index.
　ISBN 0-13-019450-6 (alk. paper)
　1. Medical assistants—Outlines, syllabi, etc.
　2. Physicians' assistangs—Outlines, syllabi etc.
　I. Hemby, Marsha Perkins. Medical assisting
review.　II. Title.
　R728.8.H46 2000
　610.73′7′076—dc21　　　　　　　00-061124

Publisher: Julie Alexander
Executive Editor: Greg Vis
Acquisitions Editors: Mark Cohen and Barbara Krawiec
Managing Development Editor: Marilyn Meserve
Director of Production and Manufacturing: Bruce Johnson
Managing Production Editor: Patrick Walsh
Production Editor: Tonia Grubb, York Production Services
Production Liaison: Danielle Newhouse
Manufacturing Manager: Ilene Sanford
Creative Director: Marianne Frasco
Cover Design Coordinator: Maria Guglielmo
Cover and Interior Designer: Janice Bielawa
Director of Marketing: Leslie Cavaliere
Marketing Coordinator: Cindy Frederick
Editorial Assistants: Melissa Kerian and Mary Ellen
　　Ruitenberg
Composition: York Production Services
Printing and Binding: The Banta Company

Prentice-Hall International (UK) Limited, *London*
Prentice-Hall of Australia Pty. Limited, *Sydney*
Prentice-Hall of Canada, Inc., *Toronto*
Prentice-Hall Hispanoamericana, S.A., *Mexico*
Prentice-Hall of India Private Limited, *New Delhi*
Prentice-Hall of Japan, Inc., *Tokyo*
Prentice-Hall Singapore Pte. Ltd.
Editora Prentice-Hall do Brasil, Ltda., *Rio de Janeiro*

Notice: The procedures described in this textbook are based on consultation with medical authorities. The author and publisher have taken care to make certain that these procedures reflect currently accepted clinical practice; however, they cannot be considered absolute recommendations.

The material in this textbook contains the most current information available at the time of publication. However, federal, state and local guidelines concerning clinical practices, including without limitation, those governing infection control and universal precautions, change rapidly. The reader should note, therefore, that new regulations may require changes in some procedures.

It is the responsibility of the reader to familarize himself or herself with the policies and procedures set by federal, state and local agencies, as well as the institution or agency where the reader is employed. The authors and the publishers of this textbook, and the supplements written to accompany it, disclaim any liability, loss or risk resulting directly or indirectly from the suggested procedures and theory, from any undetected errors, or from the reader's misunderstanding of the text. It is the reader's responsibility to stay informed of any new changes or recommendations made by any federal, state and local agency as well as by his or her employing health care institution or agency.

> *To my husband, Gene, who thinks anything is possible as long as it is for the good of the student, and who always says, "You can" when I'm thinking, "I can't."*

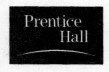

18　17　16　15　14
ISBN 0-13-019450-6

Contents

Preface

The purpose of this book is review. It serves as a study guide for the Certification and Registration Examination for Medical Assistants. The book is an effort to review briefly, but as thoroughly as possible, critical areas of medical assisting using an outline format. This format is used to obtain as much information as possible in a concise manner. The "Content Outline of the American Association of Medical Assistants' Certification Examination" has been followed so that all areas of the exam will be addressed and reviewed. The book can be used as a review prior to the certification or as a source for teaching a review course prior to the examination.

This book is composed of an introduction chapter and 19 chapters covering topics of the AAMA and RMA Content Outline. At the end of each chapter, there are questions for review and answers with explanations that should assist in study and review for the examination. There is also a CD with more than 400 questions and answers for review.

This book is a good outline format for instructors to use as a teaching guide and resource. Students can use this book in place of or in addition to note taking. High schools with health occupations classes might also use this book as a resource or a text.

Marsha Perkins Hemby

Reviewers

Barbara M. Dahl, CMA, CPC
Coordinator, Medical Assisting Program
Whatcom Community College
Bellingham, Washington

Peggy M. Krueger, RN, BSN, MEd, CMA
Program Coordinator—Medical Assistant Program
Linn-Benton Community College
Albany, Oregon

Mary Webber, MEd, CMA/RMA
Medical Assistant Program Coordinator/Instructor
Burlington County Institute of Technology
Medford, New Jersey

Introduction

 SUCCESS ACROSS THE BOARDS:
THE PRENTICE HALL HEALTH REVIEW SERIES

Prentice Hall Health is pleased to present *Success Across the Boards,* our new review series. These authoritative texts give you expert help in preparing for certifying examinations. Each title in the series comes with its own technology package, including a CD-ROM and a Companion Website. You will find that this powerful combination of text and media provides you with expert help and guidance for achieving success across the boards. This outline review for the Medical Assistant provides help for preparing for the CMA or RMA Examination.

COMPONENTS OF THE SERIES

The series is made up of two separate books and CD combinations as well as a Companion Website that supports both books.

Outline Review for the Medical Assistant by Marsha Perkins Hemby

- *About the Book:*
- *Outline Content Review:* Key topics that may be covered on the CMA or RMA examinations are included in this book. With the easy-to-use outline format, you can quickly identify the important ideas, concepts, and facts that are presented. Important terms are defined where necessary, and illustrations are included where they will help illuminate and clarify information. The concept of the review book is to make it easier to understand information you have learned elsewhere—in courses, from textbooks, in the field. The purpose of the outline format is to help you focus your review on the most important information and use your study time most effectively.
- *Key Concepts:* Be sure to scan the key concepts highlighted in the margins. These are important points to remember and will be helpful to you during your last-minute review before the exam.
- *Study Questions:* Multiple choice questions at the end of each chapter follow the format of questions that appear on the exam. Working through these questions after reviewing each chapter outline will help you assess your strengths and weaknesses in each topic of study. Correct answers and comprehensive rationales are included. All questions are referenced to related textbooks so that you can quickly and easily find resources for more in-depth explanation or study on a specific topic.

- **About the CD-ROM:** A Study Wizard CD-ROM is included in the back of this book. This CD provides additional practice multiple-choice questions, important A&P information, and an audio glossary.
- *Practice Questions:* The accompanying CD includes all questions presented in the book *plus* 200 unique questions. The software was designed so that you can practice by topic or through simulated exams. Correct answers and comprehensive rationales and references follow all questions. You will receive immediate feedback to identify your strengths and weaknesses in each topic covered.
- *Basic Anatomy Review:* This is an excellent resource featuring full-color art for quick and easy review of basic anatomy and physiology as you prepare for this critical section of the exam.
- *Audio Glossary:* Over 600 words and definitions are pronounced and will help you review the definitions and practice pronunciations of the all-important terms you need to know.

Companion Website for Medical Assisting Review

Visit the Companion Website at *www.prenhall.com/review* for additional practice, information about the exam, and links to related resources. Designed as a supplement to this book in the series, you will want to bookmark this site and return frequently for the most current information on your path to success.

Companion Book
Question and Answer Review for the Medical Assistant by Tom and Hilda Palko

Once you are comfortable with the topics on the exam and want multiple opportunities to practice your skills, this is the perfect book. The 6th edition of this best-selling review book includes over 1,800 exam-type questions with answers, comprehensive rationales, and references. By combining quick content reviews with practice questions in print, on a CD, or on the web, you will increase your likelihood of success on the exam.

CERTIFICATION

There are two national certifying agencies for the medical assisting profession recognized by the U.S. Department of Education: the American Association of Medical Assistants (AAMA) and the Registry of Medical Assistants of the American Medical Technologists (RMA/AMT).

Qualifications for the Certified Medical Assistant (CMA)

To qualify for certification as a CMA you must

1. Be a graduate of a CAHEA(Commission on Accreditation of Allied Health Education Programs)-accredited program *or*
2. Be a graduate from ABHES (Accrediting Bureau of Health Education Schools)-accredited medical assisting program with 1 year of full-time or 2 years of part-time experience in the health care field
3. Pass the Certified Medical Assistant examination administered by the AAMA Certifying Board

Qualifications for the Registered Medical Assistant (RMA)

To qualify for certification as an RMA you must

1. Be a high school graduate or equivalent
2. Graduate from a medical assistant program accredited by an organization approved by the U.S. Department of Education *or*
3. Have formal medical training in the armed forces *or*
4. Have employment as a medical assistant for 5 years with no more than 2 years as a medical assisting instructor in a postsecondary program
5. Pass the Registered Medical Assistant examination administered by the American Medical Technologists (AMT)

✓ ABOUT THE EXAMS

Certified Medical Assistant Examination

The CMA examination is a written test, administered by the AAMA Certifying Board. The tests are given twice a year, the last Friday in January and the last Saturday in June, at 200 locations throughout the United States. Deadlines for applications are March 1 for the June test and October 1 for the January test.

The examination is based on the MARDC project outline. A Candidate's Guide, CMA Certification/Recertification Examination Application, and other general information about the test may be obtained by contacting the AAMA Certifying Board at 20 North Wacker Drive, Department 77-7999, Chicago, IL 60678-7999; telephone: 312-424-3100. For additional information you may also visit the AAMA web site at *http://www.aama-ntl.org.* We strongly encourage all exam candidates to obtain a copy of the Candidate's Guide.

The CMA examination contains 300 multiple-choice questions—100 from each of the following areas: General Information, Administrative Procedures, and Clinical Procedures.

Registered Medical Assistant Examination

The RMA exam is a computerized test, administered by the AMT. The test is given throughout the year at Cogent testing center locations and may be scheduled within 3 days of application completion.

The examination is based on the Registered Medical Assistant Competency Areas Outline, which is developed by the RMA Education, Qualifications, and Standards Committee of the AMT. A Candidate's Handbook for the RMA Certification Examination, the RMA Certification Examination Overview, and an application may be obtained by contacting the Registered Medical Assistants of American Medical Technologists, 710 Higgins Road, Park Ridge, IL 60068-5765; telephone 1-800-275-1268. For additional information you may also visit the AMT website at *http://www.amtl.com.* We strongly encourage all exam candidates to obtain a copy of the Candidate's Guide.

The RMA contains 200 questions divided as follows: 42.5% general knowledge, 22.5% administrative knowledge, and 35% clinical knowledge. *Information about examinations may change, so be sure to obtain current information by contacting the examination boards.*

STUDY TIPS

Review Materials

Choose review materials that contain the information you need to study. Save time by making sure that you aren't studying anything you don't need to. For preparation before the exam, the best study preparation would be to use both the Outline Review Book and Question and Answer Review Book. Use the references in these books to easily find related textbooks if additional study is required. We strongly encourage all exam candidates to obtain a copy of the Candidate's Guide.

Set a Study Schedule

Use your time-management skills to set a schedule that will help you feel as prepared as you can be. Consider all the relevant factors—the materials you need to study; how many months, weeks, or days until the test date; and how much time you can study each day. If you establish your schedule ahead of time and write it in your date book, you will be much more likely to follow it.

Take Practice Tests

Practice as much as possible, using questions at the end of each chapter in this book along with over 2,000 more questions available in the companion Question and Answer book, the accompanying CD, and the Companion Website. These questions were designed to follow the format of questions that appear on the exam you will take, so the more you practice with these questions, the better prepared you will be on test day.

The printed practice test in the back of the *Question and Answer Review for the Medical Assistant* and the practice tests on the CDs will give you a chance to experience the exam before you actually have to take it. It will also let you know how you're doing and where you need to do better. For best results, we recommend you take a practice test 2 to 3 weeks before you are scheduled to take the actual exam. Spend the next weeks targeting those areas in which you performed poorly by reviewing the Outline and practicing additional questions in those areas.

Practice under test-like conditions—in a quiet room, with no books or notes to help you, and with a clock telling you when to quit. Try to come as close as you can to duplicating the actual test situation.

TAKING THE EXAMINATION

Prepare Physically

When taking the exam, you need to work efficiently under time pressure. If your body is tired or under stress, you might not think as clearly or perform as well as you usually do. If you can, avoid staying up all night. Get some sleep so that you can wake up rested and alert.

Eating right is also important. The best advice is to eat a light, well-balanced meal before a test. When time is short, grab a quick-energy snack such as a banana, orange juice, or a granola bar.

The Examination Site

The examination site must be located prior to the required examination time. One suggestion is to find the site and parking facilities the day before the test. Parking fee information should be obtained so that sufficient money can be taken along on the examination day.

Allow plenty of time for travel to the site in case of unexpected mishaps such as traffic snarls. During travel, think positive thoughts (e.g., "My preparation for the exam was thorough, so I'll be able to answer the questions easily"). Maintain a confident attitude to prevent unnecessary stress.

Materials

Be sure to take all required identification materials, registration forms, and any other items required by the testing organization or center. Read information and instructions supplied by the testing organizations thoroughly to be sure you have all necessary materials before the day of the exam.

Read Test Directions

Read the examination directions thoroughly! Because some board examinations have different test sections with different question formats, it is important to be aware of changes in directions. Read each set of directions completely before starting a new section of questions.

Machine-scored tests require that you use a special pencil to fill in a small box on a computerized answer sheet. Use the right pencil (usually a no. 2) and mark your answers in the correct space. Neatness counts on these tests, because the computer can misread stray pencil marks or partially erased answers. Periodically, check the answer number against the question number to make sure they match. One question skipped can cause every answer following it to be marked incorrectly.

Selecting the Right Answer

Keep in mind that only one answer is correct. First read the stem of the question with *each* possible choice provided and eliminate choices that are obvi-

ously incorrect. Be cautious about choosing the first answer that *might* be correct; all possibilities should be considered before the final choice is made; the best answer should be selected.

If a question is complicated, try to break it down into small sections that are easy to understand. Pay special attention to qualifiers such as *only, except,* etc. For example, negative words in a question can confuse your understanding of what the question asks ("Which of the following is *not...*").

Intelligent Guessing

If you don't know the answer, eliminate those answers that you know or suspect are wrong. Your goal is to narrow down your choices. Here are some questions to ask yourself:

- Is the choice accurate in its own terms? If there's an error in the choice, for example, a term that is incorrectly defined, the answer is wrong.
- Is the choice relevant? An answer may be accurate, but it may not relate to the essence of the question.
- Are there any qualifiers, such as *always, never, all, none,* or *every*? Qualifiers make it easy to find an exception that makes a choice incorrect.

Mark answers you aren't sure of and go back to them at the end of the test. Ask yourself whether you would make the same guesses again. Chances are that you will leave your answers alone, but you may notice something that will make you change your mind—a qualifier that affects meaning or a remembered fact that will enable you to answer the question without guessing.

Watch the Clock

Keep track of how much time is left and how you are progressing. Wear a watch or bring a small clock with you to the test room. A wall clock may be broken, or there may be no clock at all.

Some students are so concerned about time, that they rush through the exam and have time left over. In such situations, it's easy to leave early. The best approach, however, is to take your time. Stay until the end so that you can check your answers.

Computerized Exams

To insure that you are comfortable with the computer test format, be sure to practice on the computer, using the CD that is included in the back of this book. During the exam, check the computer screen after an answer is entered to verify that the answer appears as it was entered.

KEYS TO SUCCESS ACROSS THE BOARDS

- Study, Review, and Practice
- Keep a positive, confident attitude
- Follow all directions on the examination
- Do your best

Good luck!

*You are encouraged to visit **http://www.prenhall.com/success** for additional tips on studying, test-taking, and other keys to success. At this stage of your education and career you will find these tips helpful. Some of the study and test-taking tips were adapted from Keys to Effective Learning, Second Edition, by Carol Carter, Joyce Bishop, and Sarah Lyman Kravits.*

SECTION I

General Information

1 Medical Terms and Vocabulary

contents

I. WORD STRUCTURE

Dividing a word into its root, prefix, suffix, and combining form, and understanding each part separately will ultimately help you discover the word's definition.

A. _Root:_ the main part of the word

Example: hypo<u>gastr</u>ic: gastr- = root; gastr- means stomach

B. _Prefix:_ the first part of the word

Example: <u>hypo</u>gastric: hypo- = prefix; hypo- means below

hypogastric = below the stomach

C. _Suffix:_ the ending of the word

Example: tonsill<u>itis</u>: -itis = suffix; -itis means inflammation of

tonsillitis = inflammation of the tonsils

D. _Combining form_: a word root plus a vowel

Example: <u>cardio</u>logy: cardio- = combining form; cardio- means heart; -logy means study of

cardiology = study of the heart

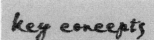

key concepts

- Difficult words can easily be defined by knowing suffix, prefix, and combining forms. Example: otorhinolaryngology—the study of ears, nose, and throat.

II. DEFINITIONS

A. Prefixes

1. Prefixes pertaining to position or placement
   a. ab- = away
   b. ad- = toward
   c. endo- = within
   d. epi- = above
   e. hyper- = above
   f. hypo- = below
   g. inter- = between
   h. retro- = behind, backward
   i. supra- = above

2. Prefixes pertaining to amounts and time
   a. bi- = two
   b. brady- = slow
   c. hemi- = half
   d. poly- = many
   e. post- = after
   f. pre- = before
   g. quadri- = four
   h. tachy- = fast
   i. tri- = three

3. Prefixes that are descriptive
   a. a- = not, negation
   b. anti- = against
   c. auto- = self
   d. dys- = difficult, painful, bad

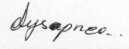
dysapnea

    e. erythro- = red
    f. hemo- = blood
    g. histo- = tissue
    h. homeo- = same, alike
    i. hydro- = water
    j. litho- = stone
    k. mal- = bad
    l. melano- = black
    m. neo- = new
    n. pseudo- = false

4. Prefixes pertaining to parts of the body
    a. adeno- = gland
    b. arthro- = joint
    c. blepharo- = eyelid
    d. cardio- = heart
    e. cervico- = neck
    f. cranio- = skull
    g. cysto- = bladder
    h. cyto- = cell
    i. dermato- = skin
    j. hepato- = liver
    k. hystero- = uterus
    l. myelo- = marrow, spinal cord

B. Suffixes

1. -algia = pain; -dynia = pain
2. -blast = not developed; -genic = forming
3. -cele = swollen sac, protrusion; -cyte = cell; -oma = tumor, growth; -lith = stone
4. -centesis = removal of fluid by puncturing
5. -cide = causing death; killing
6. -ectomy = cutting out; -tomy = cutting; -plasty = surgical repair; -rrhaphy = suturing   *-stomy : connecting 2 cavities c̄ fistula.*
7. -emesis = vomiting
8. -emia = blood condition
9. -gram = written record
10. -itis = inflammation of; -osis = diseased; -pathy = diseased; -plegia = paralysis
11. -lysis = destruction of, breaking apart; -desis = fixing together
12. -malacia = softening of; -sclerosis = hardening of
13. -megaly = enlarged
14. -mimetic = imitation
15. -opia = vision; -scopy = viewing
16. -penia = deficiency
17. -phagia = swallowing; -pnea = breathing
18. -rhea = discharge; -rhagia = bursting forth (also -rrhea, -rrhagia)

key concepts

• To define a word such as "otorhinolaryngology," break it up and define each part.
1. oto—ear   2. rhino—nose
3. laryngo—throat
4. ology—the study of
Seemingly difficult words are easy!

C. Combining forms

1. Combining forms pertaining to parts of the body
   a. angio- = vessel
   b. cephalo- = head   *cervical: neck. ; cranio: skull.*
   c. costo- = rib
   d. glosso- = tongue
   e. kerato- = cornea, horny layer ✗
   f. laparo- = abdomen
   g. myo- = muscle
   h. neuro- = nerve
   i. oculo- = eyes
   j. osteo- = bone
   k. oto- = ear
   l. phlebo- = vein
   m. pyelo- = pelvis
   n. rhino- = nose
   o. stomato- = mouth
   p. veno- = vein
2. Combining forms pertaining to organs
   a. cholecysto- = gallbladder
   b. encephalo- = brain
   c. entero- = intestines
   d. gastro- = stomach
   e. nephro- = kidney
   f. pneumo- = air in the lungs
   g. procto- = rectum
   h. pulmo- = lungs
3. Descriptive combining forms
   a. audio- = hearing
   b. chromo- = color
   c. cyano- = blue
   d. diplo- = double
   ✗ e. iatro- = related to medicine or physician
   f. leuko- = white
   g. lipo- = fat
   h. macro- = large
   i. micro- = small
   j. morpho- = shape
   k. nocto- = night
   l. oligo- = scant
   m. onco- = tumor
   n. ortho- = straight
   o. patho- = disease
   p. thrombo- = clot

III. APPLICATIONS

A. Prefixes pertaining to position or placement

1. ab- = away
   a. abrade = scrape away ✗
   b. ablation = taking away of a part ✗
2. ad- = toward
   a. adrenal = toward the kidney
   b. adduct = move a part toward the body
3. endo- = within
   a. endocarditis = inflammation within the inner lining of the heart
   b. endoscope = instrument for viewing within an organ or cavity
4. epi- = above
   a. epigastric = above the stomach
   b. epinephrine = hormone secreted by the adrenal glands above the kidney
5. hyper- = above, excessive
   a. hyperthermia = above-normal temperature
   b. hypertension = above-normal pressure
6. hypo- = below
   a. hypogastric = below the stomach
   b. hypodermic = needle injected below the skin
7. inter- = between
   a. intercostal = between the ribs
   b. interarticular = between the joints
8. retro- = behind, backward
   a. retrograde = moving or flowing backward
   b. retrolingual = behind the tongue
9. supra- = above
   a. supraorbital = above the eye's orbit
   b. suprapubic = above the pubic arch

B. Prefixes pertaining to amounts and time

1. bi- = two
   a. biceps = muscle with two heads
   b. bicuspid = having two cusps or flaps, as in the bicuspid valve of the heart
2. brady- = slow
   a. bradycardia = slow rhythm of the heart
   b. bradypnea = slow breathing
3. hemi- = half
   a. hemiplegia = paralysis of one-half of the body
   b. hemifacial = pertaining to one-half of the face
4. poly- = many
   a. polyarthritis = many inflamed joints
   b. polydactylism = extra fingers and toes

5. post- = after
    a. postoperative = after an operation
    b. postpartum = after the birth of a baby
6. pre- = before
    a. prenatal = before the birth of a baby
    b. premenstrual = before menstruation
7. quadri- = four
    a. quadriplegic = four limbs paralyzed
    b. quadriceps = muscle with four heads
8. tachy- = fast
    a. tachycardia = fast rhythm of the heart
    b. tachypnea = fast breathing
9. tri- = three
    a. triceps = muscle with three heads but one insertion
    b. tricuspid = valve between the right atrium and ventricle that has three cusps
10. baros- = weight
    a. bariatrics = branch of medicine dealing with obesity

C. Prefixes that are descriptive

1. a- = not, negation
    a. afebrile = no fever
    b. asepsis = not contaminated
2. anti- = against
    a. antibacterial = against bacteria
    b. anticoagulant = against the forming of clots
3. auto- = self
    a. autonomic = self-controlling, as in autonomic nervous system
    b. autograft = a graft of one's self
4. dys- = difficulty, painful, bad
    a. dyspnea = difficulty in breathing
    b. dyspepsia = difficulty in digesting
5. erythro- = red
    a. erythrocyte = red blood cell
    b. erythropoiesis = red blood cell formation
6. hemo- = blood
    a. hemoptysis = spitting up of blood
    b. hemolysis = destruction of blood cells
7. histo- = tissue
    a. histology = study of tissues
    b. histokinesis = movement of tissue in the body
8. homeo- = same, like
    a. homeostasis = staying the same
    b. homeoosteoplasty = grafting of bone similar to bone upon which it is grafted

9. hydro- = water
    a. hydrotherapy = treatment using water
    b. hydrocephalus = increased fluid in the brain
10. litho- = stone
    a. lithotripsy = crushing of stones
    b. lithuresis = passing of stones while urinating
11. mal- = bad
    a. malpractice = bad practice
    b. malnutrition = bad nutrition
12. melano- = black
    a. melanopathy = dark pigmentation of the skin
    b. melanglossia = black tongue
13. neo- = new
    a. neonatal = newborn
    b. neoplasm = new growing thing
14. pseudo- = false
    a. pseudotumor = symptoms like a tumor, but not a tumor
    b. pseudoplegia = paralysis of hysterical origin
15. necro- = pertaining to death or dead tissue
    a. necrosis = death of tissue
    b. necroscopy = examination of cadaver to find reason for death *(Postmortum).*
16. steno- = narrow
    a. stenosis = narrowing of a passage
    b. stenostomia = narrowing of the mouth

D. Prefixes pertaining to parts of the body

1. adeno- = gland
    a. adenoma = tumor of a gland
    b. adenitis = inflammation of a gland
2. arthro- = joint
    a. arthroplasty = plastic surgery of a joint
    b. arthrodesis = surgical fixation or fusion of a joint
3. blepharo- = eyelid
    a. blepharospasm = twitching of the eyelid
    b. blepharoptosis = drooping of the eyelid
4. cardio- = heart
    a. cardiologist = one who studies and specializes in the heart
    b. cardiogram = written record of the heart's activity
5. cervico- = neck
    a. cervicodynia = neck pain
    b. cervicofacial = pertaining to the face and neck
6. cranio- = skull
    a. craniotomy = incision into the skull
    b. craniocele = protrusion of part of the brain into the skull

7. cysto- = bladder
   a. cystoscopy = viewing and examining the bladder
   b. cystitis = inflammation of the bladder
8. cyto- = cell
   a. cytologist = one who studies cells
   b. cytogeny = formation of a cell
9. dermato- = skin
   a. dermatitis = inflammation of the skin
   b. dermatology = study of the skin
10. hepato- = liver
    a. hepatomegaly = enlarged liver
    b. hepatoma = liver tumor
11. hystero- = uterus
    a. hysterectomy = cutting out of the uterus
    b. hysterorrhexis = uterine rupture
12. myelo- = marrow, spinal cord
    a. myeloma = tumor beginning in the blood-forming part of the marrow
    b. myelopathy = disease of the spinal cord
13. cheilos- = lip
    a. cheilitis = inflamed lip
    b. cheilotomy = excision of part of the lip

E. Suffixes

1. -algia = pain; -dynia = pain
   a. neuralgia = pain along the course of a nerve
   b. myalgia = muscle tenderness and pain
   c. cephalodynia = pain in the head
   d. gastrodynia = stomach pain
2. -blast = not developed; -genic = forming
   a. erythroblast = immature red blood cell
   b. neuroblast = embryonic cell
   c. neurogenesis = forming of nerves
   d. cardiogenic = originating in the heart
3. -cele = swollen sac or protrusion; -cyte = cell; -oma = tumor
   a. cystocele = protrusion of the bladder into the vaginal wall
   b. rectocele = protrusion of the rectal wall into the vaginal wall
   c. erythrocyte = red blood cell
   d. leukocyte = white blood cell
   e. carcinoma = malignant tumor arising from epithelial tissue
   f. sarcoma = tumor arising from connective tissue
4. -centesis = removal of fluid by puncturing
   a. paracentesis = puncture of a cavity with removal of fluid
   b. arthrocentesis = removal of fluid from a joint by needle puncture

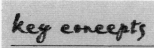

key concepts
_____

• Effectiveness in patient teaching increases when the medical assistant has a basic knowledge of surgical and diagnostic terminology.

5. -cide = causing death
   a. sporicide = spore-destroying agent
   b. bacteriocide = bacteria-destroying agent
6. -ectomy = cutting out, excision of; -tomy = cutting; -rrhaphy
   = suturing; -plasty = surgical repair; -pexy = fixation of
   a. appendectomy = cutting out of appendix
   b. hysterectomy = cutting out of uterus
   c. cystotomy = incision of bladder
   d. myotomy = dissection of muscles
   e. hysterotrachelorrhaphy = paring the edges and suturing of
      the lacerated cervix
   f. laparorrhaphy = suturing of a wound inside the abdominal
      wall
   g. pyloroplasty = surgery of the portion of the stomach that
      connects to the duodenum
   h. hernioplasty = surgical repair of a hernia
   i. cystopexy = surgical fixation of the bladder to the wall of
      abdomen
   j. nephropexy = surgical fixation of a kidney
7. -emesis = vomiting
   a. hematemesis = vomiting of blood
   b. pyemesis = vomiting of pus
8. -emia = blood condition
   a. anemia = blood condition with reduced red blood cells,
      packed cells, and hemoglobin
   b. pyemia = condition with pus-forming organisms in the
      blood
9. -gram = written record
   a. cardiogram = written record of the heart's electrical activity
   b. electroencephalogram = written record of the brain's waves
10. -itis = inflammation of; -osis = diseased; -pathy = diseased;
    -plegia = paralysis
    a. arthritis = inflammation of the joints
    b. blepharitis = inflammation of the eyelids
    c. stomatosis = any diseased condition of the mouth
    d. keratosis = diseased cornea
    e. myopathy = disease of a muscle
    f. neuropathy = disease of the nerves
    g. hemiplegia = paralysis on one side
    h. quadriplegia = paralysis of all four limbs and the trunk
11. -lysis = destruction of, breaking apart; -desis = fixing together;
    -tripsy = crushing of
    a. hemolysis = destruction of blood cells
    b. carcinolysis = destruction of cancer cells
    c. arthrodesis = surgical immobilization of a joint

d. lithotripsy = crushing of stones (calculi)

e. neurotripsy = surgical crushing of a nerve

12. -malacia = softening; -sclerosis = hardening of
   a. osteomalacia = softening of the bones
   b. neuromalacia = softening of neural tissue
   c. arteriosclerosis = hardening of the arteries
   d. otosclerosis = hardening of the bone conductors of sound in the ear

13. -megaly = enlarged
   a. splenomegaly = enlarged spleen
   b. cardiomegaly = enlarged heart

14. -mimetic = imitation
   a. sympathomimetic = imitating the sympathetic nervous system

15. -opia = vision; -scopy = viewing
   a. myopia = best vision is very close vision
   b. diplopia = double vision
   c. arthroscopy = viewing of a joint
   d. laparoscopy = viewing inside the abdominal cavity

16. -penia = deficiency
   a. thrombocytopenia = deficiency of platelets
   b. erythrocytopenia = deficiency of red blood cells

17. -phagia = swallowing; -pnea = breathing
   a. dysphagia = difficulty in swallowing
   b. dyspnea = difficulty in breathing
   c. apnea = a period of no breathing

18. -rhea = discharge; -rhagia = bursting forth (also -rrhea, -rrhagia)
   a. diarrhea = discharge or excessive flow from the bowels
   b. gastrorrhea = excessive discharge of the gastric juices
   c. hemorrhagia = bursting forth of blood
   d. metrorrhagia = bleeding from the uterus (not during normal menses)

F. Combining forms pertaining to parts of the body

1. angio- = vessel
   a. angioplasty = plastic surgery of a blood vessel
   b. angiography = radiography of blood vessels

2. cephalo- = head
   a. cephalgia = headache
   b. cephalomotor = pertaining to movement of the head

3. costo- = rib
   a. intercostal = between the ribs
   b. costectomy = resection of a rib

4. glosso- = tongue
   a. glossopharyngeal = relating to the tongue and pharynx
   b. glossopathy = disease of the tongue

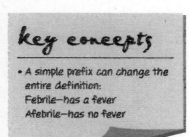

key concepts

• A simple prefix can change the entire definition:
Febrile—has a fever
Afebrile—has no fever

5. kerato- = cornea, horny layer
   a. keratotomy = incision of the cornea
   b. keratoplasty = plastic surgery of the cornea
6. laparo- = abdomen
   a. laparoscopy = viewing and examining the abdominal cavity
   b. laparorrhaphy = suturing of wounds within the abdominal wall
7. myo-= muscle
   a. myoplasty = plastic surgery of muscle tissue
   b. myoma = tumor of muscle tissue
8. neuro- = nerve
   a. neuropathy = diseased nerve
   b. neurotripsy = crushing of a nerve
9. oculo- = eyes
   a. ocular = pertaining to the eyes
   b. oculomotor = relating to eye movements
10. osteo- = bone
    a. osteomalacia = softening of a bone
    b. osteotome = cutting instrument for the bone
11. oto- = ear
    a. otoscope = instrument for viewing the ears
    b. otosclerosis = hardening of the conduction parts of the ear
12. phlebo- = vein
    a. phlebogram = tracing of venous pulse
    b. phlebitis = inflammation of a vein
13. pyelo- = pelvis
    a. pyelopathy = any disease of the kidney's pelvis
    b. pyelonephritis = inflammation of the kidney and the kidney's pelvis
14. rhino- = nose
    a. rhinoplasty = plastic surgery of the nose
    b. rhinitis = inflammation of the nose
15. stomato- = mouth
    a. stomatitis = inflammation of the mouth
    b. stomatosis = any disease of the mouth
16. veno- = vein
    a. intravenous = within the vein
    b. venation = distribution of veins in a structure

G. Combining forms pertaining to the organs
1. cholecysto- = gallbladder
   a. cholecystolithiasis = gallstones in the gallbladder
   b. cholecystectomy = cutting out the gallbladder
2. encephalo- = brain
   a. encephalitis = inflammation of the brain
   b. encephalomalacia = softening of the brain

3. entero- = intestines
   a. enterocentesis = puncture of the intestines to remove fluid
   b. enteritis = inflammation of the intestines
4. gastro- = stomach
   a. gastroenterology = study of the stomach and intestines
   b. gastrocele = hernia or protrusion of the stomach
5. nephro- = kidney
   a. nephrectomy = cutting out the kidney
   b. nephrolith = kidney stone
6. pneumo- = pertaining to respiration and air in the lungs
   a. pneumothorax = air in the pleural cavity of a lung
   b. pneumogram = record of respirations and air movement
7. procto = rectum
   a. proctoscopy = viewing of the rectum
   b. proctology = the study of the rectum
8. pulmo = lung
   a. cardiopulmonary = pertaining to the heart and lungs
   b. pulmonitis = inflammation of the lungs

H. Combining forms that are descriptive

1. audio- = hearing
   a. audiometer = machine that tests hearing
   b. audiologist = one who studies hearing
2. chromo- = color
   a. chromoturia = abnormal coloring of urine
   b. chromotherapy = using colored light as a disease treatment
3. cyano- = blue
   a. cyanosis = blue discoloration
   b. cyanopia = vision when all appears blue
4. diplo- = double
   a. diplopia = double vision
   b. diplococci = round bacteria in pairs
5. iatro- = medicine or physician related
   ятрогенческий
   a. iatrogeny = condition induced by a physician
   b. iatrotechniques = art of medicine and surgery
6. leuko- = white
   a. leukocyte = white blood cell
   b. leukoplakia = white patches on the tongue and inside the cheek
7. lipo- = fat
   a. liposuction = suctioning out of fat
   b. lipoblast = immature fat cell
8. macro- = large
   a. macromastia = abnormally large breasts
   b. macrotia = abnormally large ears

9. micro- = small
   a. microcephalus = abnormally small head
   b. microdont = having very small teeth
10. morpho- = shape
   a. morphology = study of shapes
 ✶ b. morphometry = measurement of forms
11. nocto- = night
   a. nocturia = frequent urinating at night
   b. noctiphobia = fear of the night and darkness
12. oligo- = scant, slight amount
   a. oliguria = scant amount of urine
   b. oligodipsia = abnormal decrease in the desire for fluids
13. onco- = tumor
   a. oncology = study of tumors
   b. oncogenesis = tumor formation
14. ortho- = straight, normal, correct
   a. orthopnea = cannot breathe well unless standing or sitting straight
   b. orthopedics = pertaining to the correction of deformities
15. patho- = disease
   a. pathology = study of disease
   b. pathogen = substance that is capable of producing disease
16. thrombo- = clot
   a. thrombocyte = clot-producing cell; platelet
   b. thrombolysis = destruction of a clot

IV. ABBREVIATIONS

✶ **A. Abbreviations: medication administration**
   1. a.c. = before meals
   2. ad lib = as needed
   3. A.D. = right ear
   4. A.S. = left ear
   5. A.U. = both ears, each ear
   6. b.i.d. = twice a day
   7. gtt. = drops
   8. h. = hour
   9. h.s. = bedtime, hour of sleep
   10. IM = intramuscular
   11. N.P.O. = nothing by mouth
   12. O.D. = right eye
   13. O.S. = left eye
   14. O.U. = both eyes, each eye
   15. p.c. = after meals

A. = ear

U : both (union)

O: = eye

key concepts

• Learning standard abbreviations increases efficiency in reading charts, documenting, and writing prescriptions.

16. P.O. = by mouth
17. q.d. = every day
18. q.h. = every hour
19. q.i.d. = four times a day
20. q.o.d. = every other day
21. SC = subcutaneous
22. stat. = immediately
23. t.i.d. = three times a day

B. Abbreviations: medical diagnoses

1. ASCVD = arteriosclerotic cardiovascular disease
2. CA = cancer
3. CHF = congestive heart failure
4. COPD = chronic obstructive pulmonary disease
5. CVA = cerebrovascular accident
6. DM = diabetes mellitus; IDDM = insulin-dependent diabetes mellitus; NIDDM = non-insulin-dependent diabetes mellitus
7. MI = myocardial infarction
8. MS = multiple sclerosis
9. R.A. = rheumatoid arthritis
10. TB = tuberculosis
11. TIA = transient ischemic attack
12. URI = upper respiratory infection
13. UTI = urinary tract infection

C. Miscellaneous abbreviations

1. A and W = alive and well
2. BM = bowel movement
3. BP = blood pressure
4. Bx = biopsy
5. D and C = dilation and curettage
6. DOA = dead on arrival
7. DOB = date of birth
8. Dx = diagnosis
9. ENT = ear, nose, throat
10. FU = follow-up
11. Fx = fracture
12. K = potassium
13. N/V = nausea and vomiting
14. ROS = review of systems
15. SOB = shortness of breath
16. UA = urinalysis
17. VA = visual acuity

key concepts

• Use standard abbreviations and read them in context for their meanings. Example: OD could mean right eye or overdose.

V. BODY PLANES, DIVISIONS, AND DIRECTIONS

A. *Body planes*
1. *Frontal (coronal):* divides the body into front and back (anterior and posterior); anterior = ventral, posterior = dorsal
2. *Transverse:* divides the body (at the waist) into upper and lower (superior and inferior)
3. *Midsagittal:* divides the body into right and left sides

B. *Divisions:* the abdomen is divided into four divisions with the umbilicus (navel) as the center.
1. *Right upper quadrant (RUQ):* right upper area of the abdomen; contains parts of the liver, gallbladder, and intestines.
2. *Left upper quadrant (LUQ):* left upper area of the abdomen; contains parts of the liver, stomach, pancreas, spleen, and intestines.
3. *Right lower quadrant (RLQ):* right lower area of the abdomen; contains parts of the intestines, appendix, right ureter, ovary, and fallopian tube.
4. *Left lower quadrant (LLQ):* left lower abdominal area; contains parts of the intestines, left ureter, ovary, and fallopian tube.

C. *Regions:* the abdomen is divided like a tic-tac-toe board with the umbilicus in the center.
1. *Top two side squares:* right and left hypochondriac regions
2. *Bottom two side squares:* right and left inguinal (iliac) regions
3. *Top middle square:* epigastric region
4. *Middle two side squares:* right and left lateral regions
5. *Center square:* umbilical region
6. *Lower middle square:* hypogastric region

D. Directions
1. *Distal:* at the end of a structure; the insertion of a muscle is at the distal end
2. *Proximal:* at the beginning of a structure; at the origin of a muscle
3. *Lateral:* side
4. *Medial:* middle
5. *Anterior (ventral):* front, in front of
6. *Posterior (dorsal):* back, in back of
7. *Inferior (caudal):* lower, below
8. *Superior (cephalic):* at the head, above

E. *Anatomical position:* the body is erect and standing with hands at sides, and palms forward.

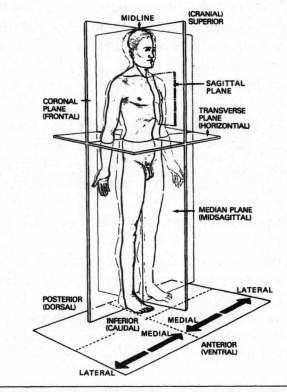

FIGURE 1–1   Anatomical direction and planes.

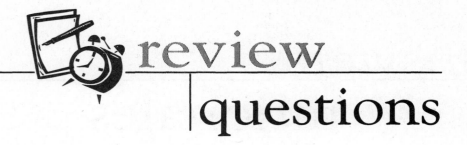

review questions

DIRECTIONS (Questions 1 through 10): Each of the numbered items or incomplete statements in this section is followed by answers or by completions of the statement. Select the ONE lettered answer or completion that is BEST in each case.

1. Otorhinolaryngology is the science of
   A. ear and throat
   B. eyes and throat
   C. eyes, ears, and nose
   D. ears, nose, and throat

2. Bariatrics is the branch of medicine dealing with
   A. skin
   B. barium swallows
   C. obesity and weight control
   D. infertility

3. Necrology is the study of
   A. removal of dead tissue
   B. mortality statistics
   C. painful deaths
   D. death caused by toxins

4. Angioplasty is
   A. changing the structure of a vessel, often by dilating
   B. softening of blood vessels
   C. rupture of a blood vessel
   D. giving medication for angina

5. A hematologist is one who studies
   A. types of hernias
   B. diagnosis and treatment of blood disorders
   C. diseases affecting only one side of the body
   D. external and internal hemorrhoids

6. Cardioversion pertains to
   A. giving a timed electric shock to the heart to obtain rhythmicity
   B. transplanting the heart of one patient into another
   C. an infant's first heartbeat after the umbilical cord is cut
   D. the QRST wave becoming arrhythmic

7. Cicatricotomy is
   A. excision of the cecum
   B. removal of wrinkles on the face
   C. incision into a scar
   D. removal of nose cilia

8. Myringotomy is
   A. excision of a tumor in the ear
   B. incision of the eardrum/tympanic membrane
   C. excision of a fungus
   D. incision into the myelin sheath

9. A cheilorrhaphy is a
   A. hemorrhage of the eyelid
   B. repair of a keloid
   C. surgical repair of a cleft lip
   D. procedure to remove toxins from the body

10. Pyloric stenosis is
    A. a constriction caused by pus
    B. narrowing of the orifice between the stomach and the duodenum
    C. pus in the urethra causing anuria
    D. narrowing of the blood vessels in the stomach

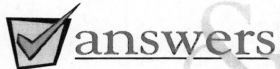

answers & rationales

1.

D Oto = ear rhino = nose laryngo = throat ology = the study of
the study of eyes = ophthalmology *(Tabers Cyclopedic Medical Dictionary)*

2.

C Baros = weight iatric = medical treatment
Dermatology = the study of skin, hair, and nails
A barium swallow is included in radiology; it is an x-ray using a contrast medium, barium.
An infertility specialist deals with infertility.
(Tabers Cyclopedic Medical Dictionary)

3.

B Necros = corpse;pertaining to death
Necrology = the study of mortality statistics
Removal of dead tissue = necrectomy
Necrotoxin = any death caused by toxins *(Tabers Cyclopedic Medical Dictionary)*

4.

A Angio = vessel plastos = molding or forming
Angioplasty is dilating a vessel for a larger passage of blood, thus oxygen-containing cells.
Angiomalacia = softening of blood vessels
Angiorrhexis = rupture of a blood vessel *(Tabers Cyclopedic Medical Dictionary)*

5.

B Heme = blood ologist = one who studies
Hernia = rupture

Hemi = half
Pathology = study of disease, thus hematopathology is the study of blood diseases
(Tabers Cyclopedic Medical Dictionary)

6.

A Cardioversion is performed for arrhythmias; giving a timed electric shock to convert the arrhythmia to a regular rhythm. *(Tabers Cyclopedic Medical Dictionary)*

7.

C Cicatrix = scar otomy = incision into *(Tabers Cyclopedic Medical Dictionary)*

8.

B Otomy = incision into myringo = tympanic membrane/eardrum *(Tabers Cyclopedic Medical Dictionary)*

9.

C Cheilo = lip rrhaphy = surgical repair of
Chelation = removal of toxins *(Tabers Cyclopedic Medical Dictionary)*

10.

B The pyloric sphincter is between the stomach and the duodenum.
Stenosis indicates narrowing. *(Tabers Cyclopedic Medical Dictionary)*

2 Anatomy and Physiology

contents

I. INTEGUMENTARY SYSTEM

For diseases of the integumentary system, one would visit the dermatologist.

A. Anatomy of the skin

1. **Epidermis:** outermost layer of the skin
2. **Dermis:** middle layer of the skin, contains:
   a. **Sweat glands:** same as sudoriferous glands: secrete sweat or sudor
   b. **Sebaceous glands:** secrete sebum, an oily, fatty substance
   c. **Nerves and nerve endings**
   d. **Blood vessels**
3. **Subcutaneous:** innermost fatty layer, the tissue below the dermis

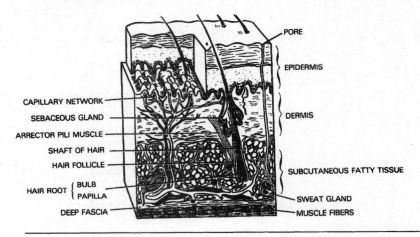

FIGURE 2-1 The integumentary system.

B. Physiology of the skin

1. **Epidermis**
   a. **Barrier from the outside:** therefore is protective
   b. Receptor for touch
   c. Preventer of water loss
2. **Dermis**
   a. **Temperature regulator:** heat escapes through blood vessel expansion and release of sweat through the pores to cool body surfaces
   b. **Sebum:** keeps skin oiled and elastic and prevents dry hair and scalp
3. **Subcutaneous**
   a. Provider for body fuel
   b. Retainer of heat
   c. Cushion for inner tissues

C. Diseases and conditions

1. **Erythema:** reddened skin
2. **Cyanosis:** blueness of the skin

3. **Jaundice:** yellowed skin
4. **Vitiligo:** white patches of the skin
5. **Acne vulgaris:** inflamed follicles of the sebaceous glands
6. **Dermatitis/eczema:** any acute or chronic skin inflammation
7. **Impetigo:** contagious skin infection usually caused by strepto-coccus or staphylococcus
8. **Psoriasis:** chronic red raised areas of the skin that are scaly and itchy; may progress into silver-yellow scales
9. **Ringworm:** fungus affecting the scalp, feet, groin, or the body in general
10. **Scabies:** infection caused by a mite that burrows under the skin, causing itching
11. **Urticaria:** hives or raised wheals caused by an allergic reaction or stress

D. Diagnostics and procedures
1. **Wood's light:** fluorescent purple light used to diagnose certain skin conditions
2. **Diascope:** flat glass plate held against the skin to examine superficial skin lesions
3. **Surgical excision and biopsy:** cutting out a lesion, mole, or skin cancer, and examining it under the microscope to identify cancerous cells
4. **Sweat chloride test:** salt content of sweat: diagnostic for cystic fibrosis

II. SKELETAL SYSTEM
For diseases of the skeletal system, one would visit the ortho-pedist; for joints, the rheumatologist.

A. Bone anatomy (approximately 206 bones)
1. **Skull:** head bone (cranium); joints of the cranium are called sutures
   a. **Frontal bone:** forehead and eye sockets
   b. **Temporal bones:** both sides around the ear and lower jaw
   c. **Parietal bones:** each side above the temporal bone
   d. **Occipital bone:** back of the head and base of the skull
2. **Scapula:** upper back bone (shoulder blade) (not to be confused with scalpel, a surgical instrument used for cutting)
3. **Clavicle:** anterior shoulder bone (collar bone)
4. **Humerus:** upper arm bone
5. **Radius:** lower arm bone on the thumb side
6. **Ulna:** lower arm bone on the little finger side
7. **Femur:** upper leg bone; longest and strongest of the bones
8. **Tibia:** lower leg bone; largest of the lower leg bones (shin bone)
9. **Fibula:** smallest of the lower leg bones; lower lateral bone of the leg

key concepts

- The skin can reveal information about the patient. Examples:
  Warmth: inflammation, fever
  Cool: lack of circulation
  Erythema (redness): inflammation
  Cyanosis (pale, blue): lack of oxygen
  Elasticity and turgor: skin hydration

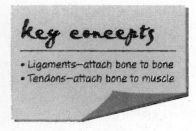

key concepts

- Ligaments—attach bone to bone
- Tendons—attach bone to muscle

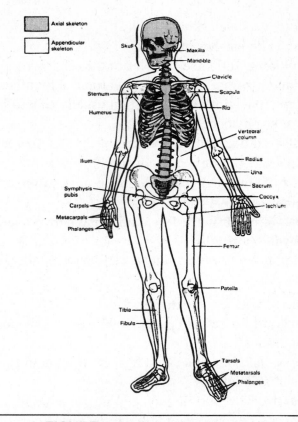

FIGURE 2-2 The skeletal system.

10. **Tarsals:** ankle bones (calcaneus is the heel bone)
11. **Metatarsals:** bones in the foot
12. **Carpals:** wrist bones
13. **Metacarpals:** hand bones
14. **Phalanges:** finger and toe bones
15. **Patella:** knee bone
16. **Sternum:** upper middle of chest; ribs connect to the sternum, and CPR chest compression is done here
    a. **Xiphoid process:** lowest portion of the sternum
17. **Vertebrae**
    C_5 a. **Cervical:** seven bones curve inward; atlas is the top bone
    T_{12} b. **Thoracic:** twelve bones curve outward
    L_5 c. **Lumbar:** five bones curve inward
    S_5 d. **Sacral:** five fused bones curve outward
    C_4 e. **Coccygeal:** four fused bones
18. **Smallest bones in body:** malleus, incus, and stapes (bones in ear) *MIS*
19. **Greater trochanter:** "knob" or muscle attachment process at the top of the femur
20. **Pelvis:** basin-shaped structure formed by the ilium, ischium, pubis, sacrum, coccyx, and ligaments

key concepts

- The smallest bones in the body are in the ear. They are the malleus, incus, and stapes, and they conduct sound waves in the ear.

B. Physiology
1. Support for the body
2. Protection of internal organs
3. Movement of the body and joints
4. Attachment for muscles
5. Formation of red blood cells in the bone marrow
6. Storage for calcium

C. Diseases and conditions
1. **Fracture:** breaking of a bone
   a. **Greenstick:** incomplete break, like a green stick
   b. **Simple:** broken bone that does not break through the skin
   c. **Compound:** broken bone that breaks through the skin
   d. **Impacted:** broken ends of the bone penetrate into each other
   e. **Spiral:** twisted break
   f. **Comminuted:** more than one piece of the bone is broken
2. **Arthritis:** inflammation of joints
3. **Gout:** painful condition usually affecting the big toe; caused by uric acid buildup
4. **Curvature of the spine:** lordosis (inward/swayback), kyphosis (outward/hunchback), and scoliosis (lateral/sideward)
5. **Sprain:** tearing of ligaments
6. **Carpal tunnel syndrome:** pressure on the median nerve in the carpal tunnel of the wrist
7. **Rickets:** lack of vitamin D, causing softening of the bones
8. **Osteoporosis:** reduction of bone mass, interfering with support
9. **Osteomalacia:** softening of bone, causing deformities, pain, and weakness

D. Diagnostics and procedures
1. **X-ray:** picture of bones to check breaks, density, and so on
2. **Laminectomy and spinal fusion:** removing part of a vertebrae in order to remove a protrusion of the disk and fusing the area to stabilize it
3. **Arthroscopy:** viewing of a joint; can also provide surgical access
4. **Arthrocentesis:** puncture, usually for removal of fluid in a joint for analysis, or for relief of pain caused by pressure
5. **Traction and reduction:** pulling on opposite ends of a bone to realign the bone

III. MUSCULAR SYSTEM

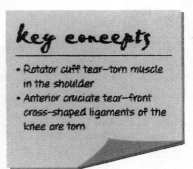

key concepts

- Rotator cuff tear—torn muscle in the shoulder
- Anterior cruciate tear—front cross-shaped ligaments of the knee are torn

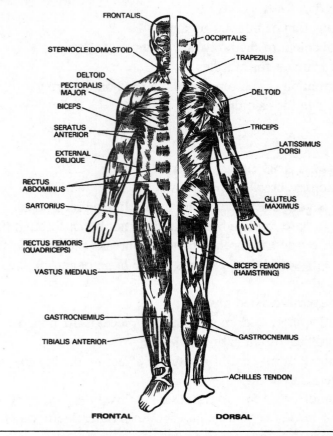

FIGURE 2-3 The muscular system.

For conditions of the muscular system, one would see an orthopedist; for therapy, a physical therapist.

A. Muscle anatomy (more than 600 muscles)

1. **Skeletal muscles:** voluntary movement; controlled by the cerebral cortex
   a. **Biceps:** upper arm bender or flexor
   b. **Triceps:** upper arm straightener or extensor
   c. **Pectoralis major:** chest muscle
   d. **Deltoid:** upper shoulder and arm muscle; site for injections
   e. **Gluteus medius:** buttocks muscle; upper outer quadrant used for injections at the dorsogluteal or ventrogluteal site
   f. **Vastus lateralis:** upper outer thigh; injection site, especially for infants
   g. **Rotator cuff muscle:** muscle that allows joint to rotate; often site of tear in shoulder
2. **Smooth muscles:** involuntary control
3. **Cardiac muscles:** automatic and rhythmic
4. **Ligaments:** attach bone to bone
   a. **Anterior cruciate:** cross-shaped ligament in knee
5. **Tendons:** attach muscle to bone

a. **Achilles tendon:** ankle; strongest tendon and site of ankle-jerk reflex

B. Muscle physiology: contraction and relaxation enabling movement

1. **Abduction:** movement away from the body
2. **Adduction:** movement toward the body

C. Diseases and conditions

1. **Tendonitis:** inflammation of the tendons
2. **Epicondylitis:** inflammation of the forearm tendon ("tennis elbow")
3. **Torticollis:** shortening of the neck muscle (sternocleidomastoid)
4. **Muscular dystrophy (MD):** wasting disease of the skeletal muscles
5. **Bursistis:** inflammation of the bursa, the fluid-filled sac that reduces friction as the joints move

D. Diagnostics and procedures

1. **Manipulation**
   a. Skillful, dextrous treatment by hand
   b. Method of examination
   c. **ROM (range of motion):** range, measured in degrees, in which a joint can be extended and flexed
   d. **PT (physical therapy):** passive movement of a joint beyond its active limit of motion
2. **X-ray:** pictures of the muscle to see abnormalities
3. **Goniometry:** measurement of the flexion of a muscle; gonio = angle

> **key concepts**
> _____
> • The intestines in sequential order:
> Small intestines:
> Duodenum, jejunum, ileum
> Large intestines:
> Ascending colon, transverse colon, descending colon, sigmoid colon, rectum, anus

IV. DIGESTIVE SYSTEM

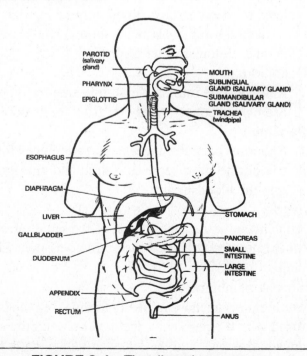

FIGURE 2-4   The digestive system.

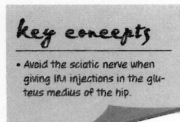

key concepts

• Avoid the sciatic nerve when giving IM injections in the gluteus medius of the hip.

For conditions of the digestive system, one would see a gastroenterologist.

A. Anatomy

1. **Mouth:** where digestion starts
2. **Pharynx:** passageway from nose and mouth to larynx and esophagus; throat
3. **Esophagus:** tube connecting the mouth and stomach
4. **Stomach:** storage and digestive area for food
5. **Small intestines**
   a. **Duodenum:** connected to the stomach by the pylorus; the first part of the small intestine
   b. **Jejunum:** second part of the small intestine
   c. **Ileum:** last portion of the small intestine
6. **Large intestines**
   a. **Cecum:** blind pouch at the beginning of the large intestine; the lower portion is the appendix
   b. **Ascending colon**
   c. **Transverse colon**
   d. **Descending colon**
   e. **Sigmoid colon**
   f. **Rectum**
   g. **Anus**
7. Accessory organs of digestion
   a. **Liver**
      1. Glycogen storer, protein manufacturer, storer of vitamin B12, and of vitamins A, D, E, K, lipid metabolizer, cholesterol manufacturer, blood volume regulator, heparin source, clotting constituent source, bile secretor, detoxifier, and biotransformer of drugs
   b. **Gallbladder**
      1. Releases bile into the small intestine for digestive aid
      2. Stores and concentrates bile from the liver
   c. **Pancreas**
      1. **Exocrine part:** produces pancreatic juices for digestion
      2. **Endocrine part:** secretes insulin and glucagon directly into the bloodstream
8. **Appendix**
   a. Attachment at the first portion of the large intestine (cecum)
   b. **McBurney's point:** site of tenderness associated with appendicitis
9. Peritoneal membrane
   a. Membrane surrounding the abdominal organs (not to be confused with the perineum, the area between the scrotum and anus in the male and the vulva and anus in the female)

10. **Visceral membranes:** cover organs
11. **Parietal membranes:** line cavities

B. Physiology

1. **Enzymes, acids, and muscle contractions** break foods down for digestion
2. **Peristalsis:** movement of food through the digestive system

C. Diseases and conditions

1. **Crohn's disease:** inflammation of the GI tract, usually the small intestine
2. **Cirrhosis:** chronic liver cell destruction
3. **Hepatitis:** inflammation of the liver; skin may be jaundiced
4. **Colitis:** inflammation of the colon
5. **Gastroenteritis:** inflammation of the stomach and intestines
6. **Hemorrhoids:** dilated, inflamed veins of the rectal mucosa
7. **Ulcers:** eating away of the mucous membrane lining
8. **Pyloric stenosis:** narrowing of the pyloric sphincter, which may prevent emptying of the contents of the stomach into the duodenum
9. **Intussusception:** the telescoping or sliding of one part of the intestine into another
10. **Hernia:** protruding of an organ through the wall of the cavity that contains it
    a. **Hiatal hernia:** stomach protruding upward into the mediastinal cavity
11. **Esophagitis:** inflammation of the esophagus caused by acid reflux

D. Diagnostics and procedures

1. **Cholecystography:** gallbladder x-ray
2. **Upper GI:** barium swallow to x-ray upper GI tract
3. **Lower GI:** barium enema to x-ray lower GI tract
4. **Colonoscopy, sigmoidoscopy, gastroscopy, proctoscopy:** viewing into specific areas of the GI tract to detect problems
5. **Hemorrhoidectomy:** excision of hemorrhoids

key concepts

• Middle ear infections should lessen as a child grows older because the eustachian tube changes from horizontal to slanting; therefore, fluid cannot pool and become infectious as easily.

V. CARDIOVASCULAR SYSTEM/LYMPHATIC SYSTEM

For diseases of the heart, one would visit a cardiologist or an internist.

1. **Heart:** pumps blood to all parts of the body
   a. **Sinoatrial node (SA node):** heart's pacemaker
   b. **Right atrium**
   c. **Tricuspid valve**
   d. **Right ventricle**
   e. **Left atrium**
   f. **Bicuspid/mitral valve**
   g. **Left ventricle:** largest chamber because of pumping action

key concepts

- According to the American Heart Association in just one to nine months after quitting smoking:
  circulation improves
  shortness of breath decreases
  energy levels increase
  cilia in lungs regrow
  infection decreases

key concepts

- Electrical conduction of the heart:
  Sinoatrial node (SA) atrioventricular node (AV) bundle of His (left and right bundle branch)
  Purkinje fibers

key concepts

- Pathway of the blood in the heart:
  Right atrium > tricuspid valve > right ventricle > pulmonary artery > lungs > pulmonary vein > left atrium > bicuspid (Mitral) valve > left ventricle > aorta > all parts of the body > back to the heart through the vena cava

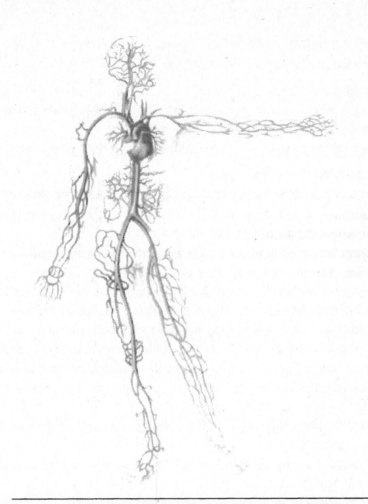

FIGURE 2-5 The cardiovascular system.

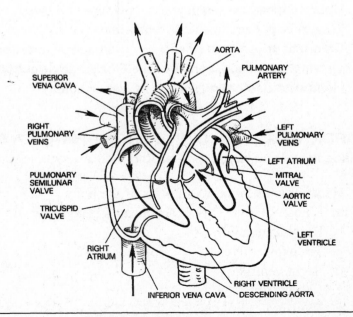

FIGURE 2-6 The heart.

2. **Arteries:** pulsate; carry blood away from the heart
   a. **Aorta:** main trunk of the arterial system; largest artery in the body
   b. **Carotid:** in the neck; check adult pulse here in CPR
   c. **Brachial:** check blood pressure here (located inside arm bend at the elbow)
   d. **Radial:** check pulse here (located inside the wrist area on the thumb side)
   e. **Femoral:** inner side of the femur; upper leg and groin area
3. **Veins:** have valves to resist backflow; carry blood back to the heart; appear dark blue
   a. **Vena cava:** principal vein draining the upper (superior vena cava) and lower (inferior vena cava) portions of the body
   b. **Median cephalic:** venipuncture vein in the middle inner arm region (inside elbow bend)
4. **Capillaries:** connect arteries and veins; for food and oxygen exchange
5. **Blood components:** most blood cells are made in the red bone marrow
   a. **Red blood cells (erythrocytes)**
      • No nucleus
      • Biconcave
      • Contain hemoglobin; carry oxygen
      • Average count: 5,000,000 per cubic millimeter ✗   *average of 2 counts and add 4 "zeros" to it.*
      • Life span: 120 days
   b. **White blood cells (leukocytes)**
      • **Agranulocytes:** lymphocytes and monocytes (<u>mononuclear</u>)
      • **Granulocytes ("polys"):** neutrophils, basophils, and eosinophils (polynuclear or multilobed)
      • Combat infections
      • Average count: 5,000 to 10,000 per cubic millimeter ✗   *average of 2 counts and <u>multiply</u> by 50*
   c. **Platelets (thrombocytes)**
      • Blood clotters
      • Average count: 200,000 to 300,000 per cubic millimeter   → *average of 2 counts and multiply by 1000.*
   d. **Plasma:** liquid portion of the blood
   e. **Serum:** fluid portion of the blood after coagulation
6. **Spleen**
   a. Production of lymphocytes
   b. Storage of red blood cells
   c. Removal of old red blood cells
7. **Lymph system:** absorbs fluid and other substances for return to the circulatory system
   a. **Lymph nodes:** lymphoid tissue along the lymph system for filtering noxious substances from the body

B. Diseases and conditions

1. **Tachycardia:** fast rhythm more than 100 beats/minute
2. **Bradycardia:** slow rhythm less than 60 beats/minute
3. **Heart block:** interruption of messages from the SA node to the atrioventricular node (AV node)
4. **Anemia:** lack of certain elements in the blood
5. **Angina pectoris:** spasm of the heart muscle because of decreased oxygen to the myocardium, causing pain and later ischemia; usually results from stress or physical activity
6. **Arteriosclerosis:** hardening of the arteries
7. **Atherosclerosis:** reduction of blood flow to the heart muscle in the myocardium because of buildup of fatty plaques in the coronary arteries, the arteries that supply the heart muscle
8. **CVA (cerebrovascular accident):** commonly known as stroke
9. **CHF (congestive heart failure):** decreased performance of the heart's pumping action
10. **Hypertension:** elevated blood pressure; usually over 140/90
11. **MI (myocardial infarction) or heart attack:** occlusion of the heart vessels causing deoxygenation and destruction of heart muscle
12. **Rheumatic heart disease:** may follow upper respiratory strep infection, causing damage to the lining of the heart and the heart valves; with mitral valve problems, patient may need prophylactic penicillin prior to surgery and dental work
13. **Mononucleosis:** increased mononuclear leukocytes in the blood; caused by Epstein–Barr virus

C. Diagnostics and procedures

1. **EKG/ECG (electrocardiogram):** tracing of the heart's rhythm
2. **Arteriogram:** x-ray of arteries
3. **Venogram:** x-ray of veins
4. **Cardiac catheterization:** visualizes heart activity and measures pressures within the heart's chambers
5. **Stress testing:** measures heart activity under controlled physical activity

VI. RESPIRATORY SYSTEM

For diseases of the respiratory system, one would visit a pulmonary or thoracic specialist or an internist.

A. Anatomy

1. **Nose:** air first enters here
2. **Larynx:** voice box
3. **Trachea (windpipe)**
4. **Lungs:** consist of bronchi, bronchioles, and alveoli; where exchange of oxygen and carbon dioxide takes place

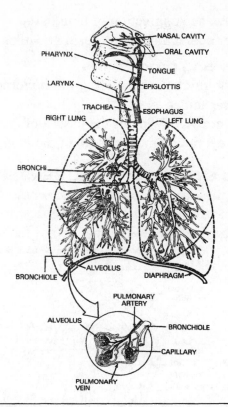

FIGURE 2-7 The respiratory system.

5. **Alveoli:** small air sacs in the lungs where carbon dioxide and oxygen exchange occurs
6. **Pleura:** serous membrane covering the lungs; has surfactant to lower surface tension

B. Physiology
1. **Exhalation:** breathing out
2. **Inhalation:** breathing in; external intercostal muscles assist with inspiration
3. Respirations are controlled by the <u>medulla oblongata in the brain</u>
4. Contractions of the diaphragm and accessory muscles cause inhalation and exhalation

C. Diseases and conditions
1. **Rhinitis:** inflammation of the nose with sneezing, watery eyes, and nasal drip
2. **Asthma:** chronic, usually allergic or infectious disorder that narrows air passages because of bronchospasms, causing wheezing or possibly severe dyspnea
3. **Bronchitis:** inflammation of the bronchi caused by narrowed bronchial airways; usually patient has cough and shortness of breath
4. **Emphysema:** enlargement of air spaces in the lungs, making exhalation difficult; usually with chronic cough and shortness of breath

5. **Pneumonia:** acute infection of lung tissue
6. **TB (tuberculosis):** infection causing nodules in the lungs

D. Diagnostics and procedures

1. **Pulmonary function tests using the spirometer:** measure various lung capacities
2. **Bronchoscopy:** viewing of the tissues of the lungs
3. **Chest x-ray:** radiological picture of the lungs

VII. NERVOUS SYSTEM/SPECIAL SENSES

For diseases of the nervous system, one would visit a neurologist.

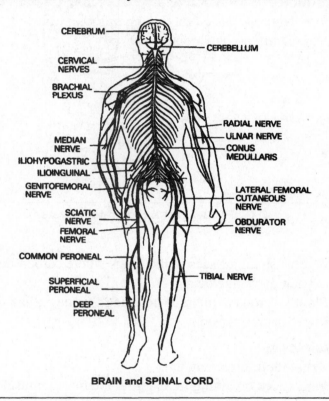

BRAIN and SPINAL CORD

FIGURE 2-8   The nervous system.

A. Anatomy

1. Peripheral nervous system and spine
   a. **Cranial nerves:** twelve pairs
   - **Olfactory:** sense of smell
   - **Optic:** vision
   - **Oculomotor:** eye movements, accommodation, and sensory perception
   - **Trochlear:** muscle sense and eye movement
   - **Trigeminal:** sensory perception for parts of the eye, nose, forehead, cheek, chin, and so on
   - **Abducens:** eye motion (problems with the abducens nerve = diplopia)

Superior oblique - CN₄.
Lateral rectus - CN₆

S₄ L₆

- **Facial:** expressions of the face, taste (problems with the facial nerve = Bell's palsy)
- **Vestibulocochlear (auditory, acoustic):** hearing and equilibrium
- **Glossopharyngeal:** taste, swallowing
- **Vagus:** coughing, sneezing, swallowing, hunger, and peristalsis
- **Accessory:** neck muscle movement
- **Hypoglossal:** tongue movements

b. **Motor (movement) and sensory (senses) nerves 31 pairs:**
  - **Neuron:** basic functioning unit of a nerve
  - **Synapse:** junction of neurons
  - **Dermatomes:** body areas enervated by nerves

c. **Autonomic nervous system:** controls involuntary functions such as heartbeat, breathing, and digestion
  - **Sympathetic:** speeds up involuntary muscle action → *fight & flight*
  - **Parasympathetic:** slows down involuntary muscle action

d. **Meninges:** coverings that protect the spinal cord and brain
  - **Dura mater:** outer
  - **Arachnoid:** middle
  - **Pia mater:** innermost

e. **Cerebrospinal fluid:** cushions the brain and spinal cord, and provides nutrients; an important part of pressure regulation in the brain

2. Central nervous system

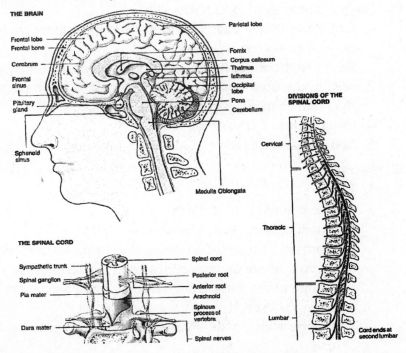

FIGURE 2-9   The brain and spinal cord.

    a. Brain
- **Cerebrum:** largest area; sensory and motor activity; intellect
- **Cerebellum:** smooth muscle movement and coordination
- **Medulla oblongata:** vital control center influencing heart-beat, breathing, and temperature
- **Pons:** influences breathing and is a reflex center
- **Midbrain:** reflex center
- **Hypothalmus:** regulates hormones, controls temperature, is the waking center, and controls appetite and sex drive
- **Convolutions (gyri):** folds in the brain

B. Physiology
1. Controls voluntary and involuntary functions, emotions, intellect, and senses

C. Diseases and conditions
1. **Encephalitis:** severe inflammation of the brain
2. **Meningitis:** inflammation of the covering of the brain and spinal cord
3. **Hydrocephalus:** excessive fluid within the brain
4. **Cerebral palsy:** brain damage before or during birth resulting in spasticity, underdevelopment, seizures, or mental retardation
5. **Herpes zoster (shingles):** inflammation along a nerve caused by the varicella virus
6. **Multiple sclerosis:** destruction of the myelin sheath, causing episodic tremors, weakness, mood swings, and vision changes

D. Diagnostics and procedures
1. **CAT scan of the brain (computerized axial tomography):** x-rays of the layers of the brain
2. **EEG (electroencephalogram):** recording of the brain waves
3. **MRI of the brain (magnetic resonance imaging):** pictures of the brain using magnetic waves
4. **Skull series:** x-rays of the brain
5. **Lumbar puncture:** cerebrospinal fluid is aspirated for examination

E. Senses
1. Eye
    a. **Iris:** colored part of the eye
    b. **Pupil:** opening that constricts or dilates
    c. **Cornea:** transparent covering of the anterior part of the eye
    d. **Retina:** where an image focuses; inner layer of the eye
    e. **Conjunctiva:** transparent covering lining the eyelids and covering the eyeball
    f. **Sclera:** white, outer layer of the eye, just under the conjunctiva
    g. **Choroid:** middle, vascular layer of the inside of the eye

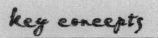

key concepts

- For CMA status:
  National Center for
  Competency Testing (NCCT)
  4352 West 107th Street
  Overland Park, KS 66207

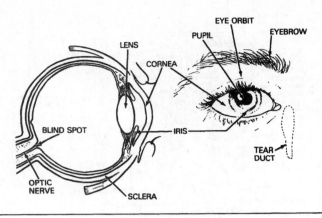

FIGURE 2-10 The eye.

h. **Lens:** transparent biconcave body that helps focus light on the retina

i. Disorders
   - **Myopia:** ability to see near objects; nearsightedness
   - **Hyperopia:** ability to see far objects; farsightedness
   - **Presbyopia:** loss of accommodation (ability to adjust near to far, and far to near) due to age
   - **Cataract:** cloudiness of the lens
   - **Glaucoma:** increased pressure on the optic nerve inside the eye; checked by using a tonometer
   - **Conjunctivitis:** inflammation of the lining of the lids

j. Diagnostics and procedures
   - **Refraction:** checking for visual correction or glasses
   - **Tonometry:** measuring intraocular pressure to check for glaucoma
   - **Visual acuity:** evaluating distance vision using the Snellen eye chart or evaluating near vision using the near vision acuity chart or often, any type of everyday reading material, such as a telephone book and newspaper
   - **Ishihara method:** checking color vision
   - **Corneal transplants**

2. Ear
   a. **Tympanic membrane:** eardrum
   b. **Middle ear:** malleus, incus, stapes (bones that conduct sound)
   c. **Eustachian tube:** connects the ear to the throat (transfer of infections from the nose and throat to the ears occurs here; as children grow, this tube slants, resulting in less transfer of infection)
   d. **Inner ear (cochlea):** contains sensory nerves for hearing and semicircular canals for balance

key concepts

- For RMA status:
  American Medical Technologies
  710 Higgins Road
  Park Ridge, IL 60068-5765

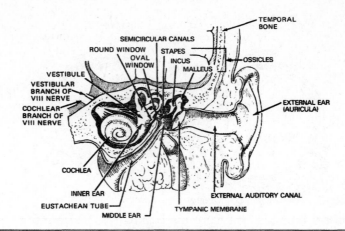

FIGURE 2-11 The ear.

e. Disorders
- **Cerumen (wax) obstruction**
- **Otitis externa (swimmer's ear)** : infection of the outer ear or otitis media (middle ear infection)
- **Ménière's disease:** dizziness (vertigo), tinnitus (ringing), and nerve loss
- **Otosclerosis:** hardening of the oval window resulting in ankylosis of the stapes

f. Diagnostics and procedures
- **Audiometry:** evaluation of hearing
- **Myringotomy:** incision of the tympanic membrane

VIII. URINARY SYSTEM

For diseases of the urinary tract or problems with the male reproductive system one would see a urologist.

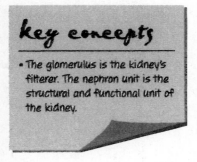

key concepts

• The glomerulus is the kidney's filterer. The nephron unit is the structural and functional unit of the kidney.

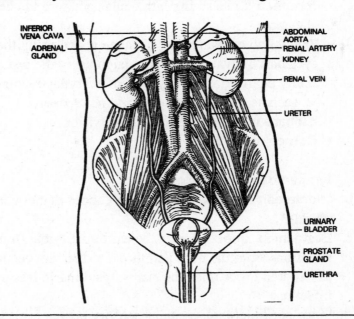

FIGURE 2-12 The urinary system.

A. Anatomy

1. **Kidneys** (two)
   a. **Nephron:** most of the work is done here
   b. **Glomerulus:** filterer
   c. **Bowman's capsule:** surrounds glomerulus
   d. **Collecting tubules:** urine is concentrated here
   e. **Renal pelvis:** holding basin for urine until passage into the ureters
2. **Ureters:** one per kidney, connecting the kidney to the bladder
3. **Bladder:** reservoir for urine
4. **Urethra:** tube leading from the bladder to the outside

B. Physiology

1. Urinary system serves to filter wastes from the body and eliminate them in the form of urine

C. Diseases and conditions

1. **Cystitis:** inflammation of the bladder
2. **Glomerulonephritis:** inflammation of the glomerulus or filterer of the kidney
3. **Renal failure:** cessation of kidney function
4. **Renal calculi (kidney stones):** stone mass or masses present in the pelvis of the kidney
5. **Incontinence:** inability to retain urine (or feces) because of loss of muscle sphincter control

D. Diagnostics and procedures

1. **Cystoscopy:** viewing of the bladder
2. **Urinalysis and 24-hour collections:** analysis of the urine physically and chemically or collection to check the amount of output
3. **IVP (intravenous pyelography):** x-rays of the urinary tract
4. **Dialysis:** mechanical removal of waste products from the blood
5. **Transplants:** replacement of a nonfunctioning kidney with a kidney from a donor

key concepts

- The fallopian tubes are the most frequent site of ectopic pregnancies.

IX. REPRODUCTIVE SYSTEM

For problems of the female reproductive system, one would see a gynecologist; if pregnant, an obstetrician. The male would see a urologist.

A. Female anatomy

1. **Ovaries (two):** primary reproductive organs
2. **Fallopian tubes:** next to the ovaries and connecting to the uterus
3. **Uterus:** normally hollow muscular organ
   a. **Cervix:** the lower opening into the uterus
4. **Vagina:** opening from the outside of body connecting to the cervix
5. **Breasts:** mammary glands

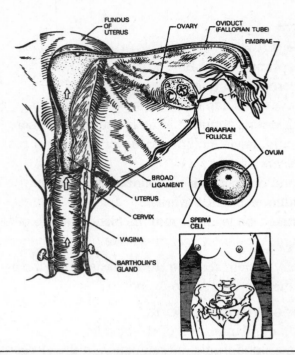

FIGURE 2-13   The female reproductive system.

B. Male anatomy

1. **Testes:** primary sex organs of the male; suspended in the scrotum
2. **Penis:** male organ of copulation/urination
3. **Prostate gland:** muscular secreting tissue surrounding the urethra

C. Female physiology

1. **Ovaries:** for development of eggs or ova and estrogen secretion
2. **Uterine lining or endometrium:** builds up to prepare for implantation of fertilized ovum or for shedding, as in menstruation
3. **Breasts:** for milk production

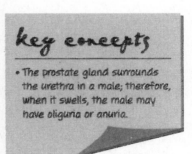

key concepts

• The prostate gland surrounds the urethra in a male; therefore, when it swells, the male may have oliguria or anuria.

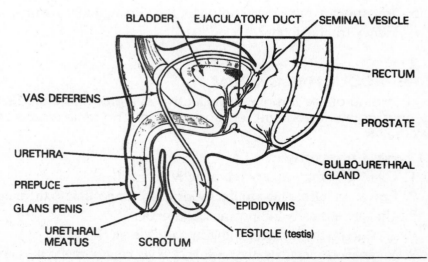

FIGURE 2-14   The male reproductive system.

D. Male physiology

1. **Testes:** produce sperm and secrete testosterone
2. **Penis:** has within it the urethra, a tube for expelling semen or urine
3. **Prostate:** contracts during ejaculation and secretes part of the seminal fluid

E. Diseases and conditions

1. **Hydrocele:** excessive fluid in the scrotum of the male
2. **Prostatic hypertrophy:** enlargement of the prostate gland
3. **Prostatectomy:** excision of the prostate gland
4. **Endometriosis:** endometrium-like tissue found in abnormal places, usually the pelvic area
5. **Hysterectomy:** cutting out of the uterus
6. **Mastectomy:** removal of the breast due to cancer
7. **STD (sexually transmitted diseases):** AIDS, syphilis, gonorrhea, chlamydial infections, trichomoniasis, genital herpes
8. **Ectopic pregnancy:** implantation of a fertilized ova somewhere other than the uterus, usually the fallopian tubes
9. **Prostatitis:** inflammation of the prostate gland
10. **Vaginitis:** inflammation of the vagina caused by yeast, bacteria, or other organisms
11. **Impotence:** inability to achieve or maintain erection of the penis

TORCH.

F. Diagnostics and procedures

1. Testicular self-examination
   a. Testicles rolled gently between thumb and forefingers of both hands
   b. Lumps or knots reported to a doctor
2. Breast self-examination
   a. Breasts rubbed in shower with flat fingers (not fingertips) to feel for lumps (circling breasts, inside out)
   b. Reflection in mirror: hands by side, then over head; look for asymmetry, dimpling, swelling, or nipple changes
   c. Supine: circle breasts inside out again with flat fingers; check nipples for discharge by gently squeezing
3. **Pap smear:** obtaining microscopic samples of the cervical area to check for abnormal cells
4. **Mammogram:** x-ray of the breasts
5. **D and C (dilation and curettage):** scraping of the inside of the uterus
6. **Cryotherapy or cauterization:** freeze or burn therapy
7. **Amniocentesis:** puncture of the amniotic sac to remove fluid for study

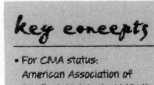

key concepts

• For CMA status:
American Association of
Medical Assistants (AAMA)
20 North Wacker Drive
Suite 1575
Chicago, IL 60606-2903

X. ENDOCRINE SYSTEM

For diseases of the endocrine system, one would see an endocrinologist.

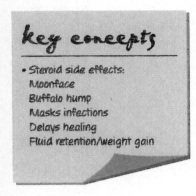

key concepts

• Steroid side effects:
  Moonface
  Buffalo hump
  Masks infections
  Delays healing
  Fluid retention/weight gain

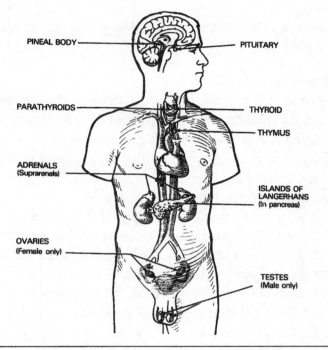

FIGURE 2-15   The endocrine system.

A. Anatomy

1. **Pituitary gland:** located at the base of the brain (called "master gland")
   a. Anterior lobe hormones
      • Growth hormone
      • Prolactin
      • Thyroid-stimulating hormone
      • Adrenocorticotropic hormone
      • Follicle-stimulating hormone
      • Luteinizing hormone
   b. Posterior lobe hormones
      • Antidiuretic hormone   (vasopressin .
      • Oxytocin
2. **Thyroid gland:** located in the anterior part of the neck
   a. Thyroxine
   b. Triiodothyronine
   c. Calcitonin
3. **Adrenal gland:** located at the top of each kidney
   a. Adrenal medulla hormones
      • Epinephrine
      • Norepinephrine

   b. Adrenal cortex hormones
      • Aldosterone
      • Glucocorticoids/cortisol
      • Androgens or sex hormones
4. **Parathyroid:** located on the posterior surface of the thyroid gland
   a. Parathormone
5. **Pancreas:** located behind the stomach
   a. Islets (Islands) of Langerhans
      • Insulin
      • Glucagon
6. **Pineal gland:** located in third ventricle of the brain
   a. Melatonin
7. **Thymus:** located behind the sternum
   a. Thymosin
8. **Reproductive glands**
   a. **Ovaries:** located in the female pelvis
      • Estrogen
      • Progesterone
   b. **Testes:** located in the male scrotum
      • Testosterone

key concepts

• The pituitary gland is the master gland, because it controls and signals all other glands.

B. Physiology

1. **Pituitary:** secretions controlled by the hypothalamus
   a. **Growth hormone:** stimulates cell growth and reproduction
   b. **Prolactin:** promotes female breast development and milk production and stimulates male sex hormone production
   c. **Thyroid-stimulating hormone:** controls secretion of the thyroid gland's hormones
   d. **Adrenocorticotropic hormone:** controls secretion of certain hormones from the adrenal cortex
   e. **Follicle-stimulating hormone:** influences the reproductive organs
   f. **Antidiuretic hormone:** reduces excretion of the kidneys, sometimes affects blood pressure
   g. **Oxytocin:** causes uterine contractions and influences milk production
2. **Thyroid:** removes iodine from the blood
   a. **Thyroxine and triiodothyronine:** influences metabolism, protein synthesis, and maturation of the nervous system
   b. **Calcitonin:** decreases blood calcium and phosphate levels
3. **Adrenals**
   a. **Epinephrine:** like sympathetic nervous system, increases heart rate; is a vasoconstrictor and thus increases blood pressure; is a bronchiole relaxer

b. **Aldosterone:** helps conserve sodium and water in the kidneys and decreases potassium reabsorption

c. **Glucocorticoids:** influence protein, fat, and glucose metabolism, therefore influencing blood glucose; also serve as anti-inflammatories

d. **Sex hormones:** promote sex characteristics and functions

4. **Parathyroid glands**

a. **Parathormone:** increases blood calcium and decreases blood phosphate

5. **Pancreas**

a. **Insulin:** increases metabolism of carbohydrates; decreases blood sugar

b. **Glucagon:** stimulates release of glycogen from the liver promoting increased blood sugar

6. **Pineal**

a. **Melatonin:** appears to decrease reproductive activities by inhibiting gonadotropic hormones

7. **Thymus**

a. **Thymosin:** affects lymphocyte production

8. **Reproductive glands**

a. **Estrogen, progesterone and testosterone:** promote sexual characteristics and functions

C. Diseases and conditions

1. **Dwarfism:** lack of growth hormone; if during childhood, called cretinism

2. **Gigantism:** excess of growth hormone in childhood

3. **Acromegaly:** excess of growth hormone in adulthood

4. **Hypothyroidism:** decrease in thyroid hormone production, and thus a decrease in metabolic rate; called myxedema in adulthood

5. **Hyperthyroidism:** excess of thyroid hormone production, and thus an increase in metabolic rate; Graves' disease

a. **Exophthalmia:** bulging eyes

b. **Goiter:** enlarged thyroid gland because of a lack of iodine

6. **Tetany:** uncontrolled twitching of the muscles because of hypoparathyroidism

7. **Cushing's disease:** excess of glucocorticoids causing edema of the face and fatty tissue on the back ("moonface" and "buffalo hump")

8. **Diabetes mellitus:** high blood sugar and sugar in the urine because of a lack of insulin

D. Diagnostics and procedures

1. **Thyroidectomy:** surgical removal of the thyroid gland

2. **Thyroid function tests:** check function of the thyroid gland

3. **Thyroid scan:** checks thyroid's absorption ability

4. **Glucose tolerance test:** checks patient's metabolism of glucose; confirmatory test for diabetes

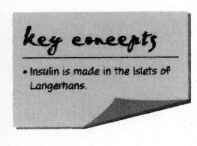

key concepts

• Insulin is made in the Islets of Langerhans.

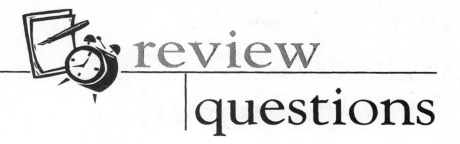

review questions

DIRECTIONS (Questions 1 through 10): Each of the numbered items or incomplete statements in this section is followed by answers or by completions of the statement. Select the ONE lettered answer or completion that is BEST in each case.

1. What portion of the skin includes the blood vessels and nerve endings?
   A. epidermis
   B. dermis
   C. subcutaneous
   D. arrector pili

2. Which bone is between the patella and the tarsals?
   A. clavicle
   B. ulna
   C. metatarsals
   D. tibia

3. The carpals are part of the
   A. wrist
   B. ankle
   C. skull
   D. fingers

4. A painful condition due to uric acid buildup that often affects the big toe is
   A. ringworm
   B. gout
   C. osteomalacia
   D. urticaria

5. Shortening of the sternocleidomastoid muscle is
   A. epicondylitis
   B. torticollis
   C. cervicitis
   D. otitis media

6. The cecum is attached to the
   A. ascending colon
   B. transverse colon
   C. descending colon
   D. sigmoid colon

7. Check the following for tenderness gives a clue for the diagnosis of appendicitis
   A. Babinski reflex
   B. Ortolani's point
   C. McBurney's point
   D. Trousseau's sign

8. The assessment of NSR means that the patient has
   A. a heart murmur
   B. cardiomegaly
   C. a normal heartbeat
   D. bradycardia generated only by the AV node

9. The fluid portion of blood after coagulation is
   A. serum
   B. plasma
   C. lymph
   D. erythrocytes

10. For diseases of the integumentary system one would see a/an
    A. orthopedist
    B. urologist
    C. endocrinologist
    D. dermatologist

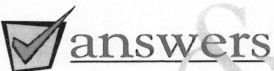

answers & rationales

1.

B. Blood vessels and nerve endings are in the dermis only. The epidermis is the outer layer of skin. The subcutaneous layer is the fatty portion, and the arrector pili are muscle fibers that make the hair "stand on end." *(Frazier, p 114)*

2.

D. The tibia and the fibula are between the patella (kneecap) and the tarsals (ankle bones). The clavicle is the collar bone; the ulna is the bone beside the radius in the lower arm; the metatarsals are the foot bones. *(Frazier, p 114)*

3.

A. The carpals are the wrist bones; the ankle bones are the tarsals; there are many skull bones; the finger and toe bones are the phalanges. *(Frazier, p 114)*

4.

B. Gout is caused by uric acid buildup and often affects the big toe. Ringworm can be anywhere on the body; osteomalacia is the softening of bones; urticaria is a rash or hives. *(Frazier, p 156)*

5.

B. Torticollis is shortening of the sternocleidomastoid muscle. Epicondylitis is an inflamed epicondyle of the humerus; cervicitis is inflammation of the cervix; otitis media is middle ear infection. *(Tabers Cyclopedic Medical Dictionary)*

6.

A. The cecum is part of the ascending colon where the appendix is attached. *(Frazier, p 188)*

7.

C. Tenderness at McBurney's point is a clue to appendicitis. It is located between the umbilicus and the top of the iliac spine on the right. A positive Babinski reflex shows a neurological deficit unless in a newborn. Ortolani's sign indicates dislocation of the hip in infants. Trousseau's sign indicates tetany. *(Frazier, p 188)*

8.

C. A normal heartbeat is described as NSR or normal sinus rhythm. *(self)*

9.

A. The fluid portion of blood after it has clotted is the serum. Plasma is the fluid portion of the blood before coagulation. Lymph is colorless and may contain fats, proteins, and lymphocytes. Erythrocytes are part of the solid components of blood—the red blood cells. *(Estridge, pp 185–87)*

10.

D. Dermatologist. An orthopedist is seen for diseases of the skeletal system; a urologist is seen for diseases of the urinary system or the male reproductive system; an endocrinologist is seen for diseases of the endocrine system. *(self)*

CHAPTER

3 Professionalism

contents

I. PROFESSIONAL BEHAVIOR AND TRAITS

A. Desirable qualities

1. Intelligence
2. Friendliness
3. Empathy
4. Punctuality
5. Maintenance of good health and hygiene
6. Membership in professional organizations
7. Currency of knowledge and continued reading of literature pertaining to the field of medical assisting
8. Knowledge of the scope of practice and the limitations of practice within that scope
9. Cooperative team membership
10. Maintenance of poise and self-control
11. Self-motivation
12. Good attitude and positive outlook
    a. No taking part in office gossip
    b. No breaches of confidentiality
    c. Admitting one's errors
    d. Loyalty to office and employer
    e. Customer-oriented
13. No use of profanity
14. No gum chewing or eating during patient communication
15. Proper English usage and good communication skills

B. Professional dress

1. Conservative and business-like
2. Conservative necklines and hemlines
3. Clean, wrinkle-free clothes and polished shoes
4. Clean breath and clean smell (remember that some people are allergic to perfumes)
5. Fingernails and hair conservative in color and length
6. No tattoos or body piercing other than conservative ear piercing
7. No tight, body-hugging clothes or panties or panty-lines showing
8. Good oral hygiene
9. No odors caused by smoking

C. Appearance of office should be orderly and clean.

II. JOB DESCRIPTION

A. Medical Assistant

1. Professional and multiskilled
2. Dedicated to assisting in all aspects of medical assisting practice under a physician

3. Patient caregiver
4. Skilled in clinical, administrative, and laboratory procedures
5. Capable at managerial and supervisory roles
6. Good communication skills
7. Adheres to ethical and legal practices
8. Skilled in emergency management

III. PROFESSIONAL ORGANIZATIONS
Membership is a must!

A. AAMA: American Association of Medical Assistants
1. Journal: **The Professional Medical Assistant** or **PMA**
2. Certification awarded to those passing the national examination
3. Recertification every five years; 60 recertification points needed (20 general, 20 administrative, and 20 clinical including 15 overall AAMA CEUs)
4. Local AAMA chapter membership and state MA society membership when joining national organization
   a. Continuing education by attending meetings and seminars, study courses through AAMA or **PMA,** college courses, and authorship

B. AAMT: American Association of Medical Transcriptionists
1. Bimonthly newsletter and quarterly journal
2. Voluntary certification by examination
3. Recertification every three years; 30 CEUs needed

C. RMA: Registered Medical Assistants
1. Establishment by American Medical Technologists (AMT)
2. Certification by examination
3. Revalidation every five years

D. PSI: Professional Secretaries International, CPS: certified professional secretary
1. Examination and work requirements for certification
2. Two-day examination twice a year

E. NCCT-tested medical assistant needs to recertify every five years with seven CEUs
(Information subject to change; see Study Tips, p. xiii at beginning of book)

IV. CONTINUING EDUCATION

A. CEUs (continuing education units) obtained in many ways
1. Program credit at local, state, and national meetings
2. Workshops approved by each organization

key concepts

• Five components of the AAMA Code of Ethics include:
1. Render service with full respect for the dignity of humanity. Respect confidential information obtained through employment unless legally authorized or required by responsible performance of duty to divulge such information.
2. Uphold the honor and high principles of the profession and accept its disciplines.
3. Seek to continually improve the knowledge and skills of medical assistants for the benefit of patients and professional colleagues.
4. Participate in additional service activities aimed toward improving the health and well-being of the community.

key concepts

• Being intelligent without a good attitude is really playing dumb!

key concepts

• Leave "honey" to the bees and "sweetheart" to your mate. Patients should be addressed by their names. Ex. Mrs. Smith

3. Tests following articles in professional magazines

4. Guided study programs through the mail

V. ETHICS

A. AAMA Code of Ethics

1. **Dignity of the patient:** maintained with all patients regardless of circumstances

2. **Confidentiality:** practiced in all areas concerning patients

3. **Professionalism:** practiced at all times

4. **Continuing education:** pursued for professional growth

5. **Good citizenship:** observed by participation in community affairs

6. Medical Assistants may obtain a copy of *"Current Opinions of Ethical and Judicial Affairs"* published by the AMA for ethical guidelines

VI. QUALITY ASSURANCE AND RISK MANAGEMENT

A. Monitoring and evaluating systems in place

B. Standards of quality established and practiced

C. Accreditation of all areas utilized for continued self-assessment

D. Safety promotion in all areas; risks identified and improved

E. Lack of quality care or practices identified and improved

F. Liabilities reduced; liability insurance in needed areas

G. Possible risks to assess in every office

1. Needle sticks

2. Patient allergies

3. Patient specimen mix-ups

4. Writing in wrong chart

5. Drug errors especially due to similar spelling and sound

6. Mercury thermometer spills

7. Loss of computer information if not saved or backed up

8. Drug sample expiration dates

9. Prescription pad visibility

10. Waste management

11. In-house narcotics

12. No material safety data sheets (MSDS)

13. Not editing after computer input

key concepts

- Be sure to enunciate words and document them clearly or the definition could be the opposite. Example: hypoglycemia hyperglycemia

key concepts

MEDICAL ASSISTANT CREED
- I believe in the principles and purposes of the profession of medical assisting.
- I endeavor to be more effective.
- I aspire to render greater service.
- I protect the confidence entrusted to me.
- I am loyal to my employer.
- I am true to the ethics of my profession.
- I am strengthened by compassion, courage, and faith.
- I am dedicated to the care and well-being of all patients.

H. Some quality processes

1. Call to remind patients of appointments
2. Update data every visit
3. Doctor signs progress notes, lab reports, etc., prior to filing chart
4. Keep log of patients who have outside diagnostic tests done
5. Call patients 4 hours to 1 day following surgery to check up on them
6. Monitor patient flow so no patient has to wait more than 15–20 minutes
7. Survey patients for office and employee evaluation
8. Wash hands in front of patients
9. Encourage neatness and good manners
10. Keep restrooms clean and well-stocked

key concepts

- Listening is often more therapeutic than giving advice.

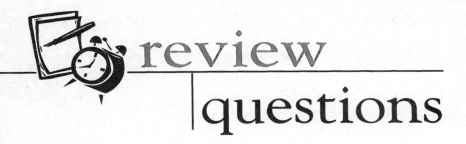
DIRECTIONS (Questions 1 through 10): Each of the numbered items or incomplete statements in this section is followed by answers or by completions of the statement. Select the ONE lettered answer or completion that is BEST in each case.

1. You are at the front desk. A patient arrives and begins arguing about his bill. Your best action is to
   A. tell him you didn't make the mistake, but you will find out who did
   B. tell him to calm down and have a seat
   C. apologize for the error and take the patient to the billing clerk to correct it
   D. tell the patient you will listen to him only when he gets quiet

2. Your supervisor tells you it is unprofessional to wear the denim skirt you have on. Your best action is to
   A. Tell her they let you wear it at the last place you worked
   B. tell her you see nothing wrong with it; clothes make you neither professional or unprofessional
   C. tell her Janie was wearing one just like it last week
   D. ask if you will need to go home and change to something else

3. You have finished getting your doctor's patients' vital signs, weight, and height. You notice Janie is behind on her doctor's patients. Your best action is to
   A. take a break so you'll be ready for the next hour

   B. look at the schedule to see if there is something you can do to get ahead of schedule
   C. ask Janie if she would like for you to help her check vital signs, height, and weight
   D. tell Janie's doctor she is behind and ask him if he would like your help

4. You want to be a safe and accurate professional. Every time you check blood pressures you
   A. ask Janie to recheck them
   B. check them twice; once in the right arm and once in the left arm
   C. document the blood pressure in the chart, rechecking when the reading is markedly different from the last visit
   D. ask the doctor if the reading sounds right to him

5. You made an error in documenting. Your best action is to
   A. white it out and correct it
   B. mark a line through the error, date and initial it
   C. correct the error, but do not initial it so no one will blame you for the error
   D. copy the page while correcting the error

6. You were filing insurance and found out a former classmate, Mary, is pregnant. Your best action is to

A. ask the receptionist if Mary is married now

B. call Mary and congratulate her

C. say nothing unless Mary tells you that she is pregnant

D. congratulate Mary and her husband the next day when you bump into them

7. Your doctor is being sued. When a patient asks about the suit, you say

A. "Who told you about it?"

B. "I'm sorry but any information about whether or not he is being sued would be confidential."

C. "It really is none of my business."

D. "You realize this day and time people can be sued for anything!"

8. You have passed the AAMA national exam for medical assisting and are now certified. You are especially relieved because you know that

A. you are now certified for life

B. you will never have to listen to another lecture

C. you may not have to take the exam again if you obtain CEUs

D. even though you must take the exam again periodically, it will be at least a few years

9. Your doctor has a tendency to lose his temper and curse on occasion. When asked by a potential employee "How is it to work with Dr. Smith?" you respond

A. "Oh, he curses occasionally, but he is a good employer."

B. "I don't like it when he loses his temper and curses, but I need this job."

C. "I would rather not prejudice you one way or the other since everybody has different viewpoints."

D. "I'd rather not answer that."

10. You want to be festive at the office during the holiday season. Your best action is to

A. wear underwear with Santas on them so they will shine through your white uniform

B. apply artificial nails with holly and berries painted on them

C. wear a pine-scented holiday perfume

D. Wear small conservative Santa earrings

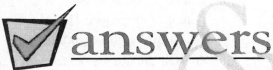
answers
rationales

1.

C. You are a representative of all parts of the office, so it is a good idea to apologize whether you made the mistake or not. You want to get a dissatisfied patient out of the waiting room and into a private area to voice his grievances. Telling someone to calm down usually makes matters worse. Telling the patient you will listen only when he gets quiet may make the patient even madder and very defensive. *(Milliken, p 267)*

2.

D. Your supervisor is someone who can tell you what to wear and what not to wear according to office policy. They may even be able to fire you, so it is best to adhere to the office dress code. It doesn't matter that you could wear denim where you worked before, because each office may have different dress codes. Whether denim has been worn by someone else is irrelevant, because at this point in time, the supervisor is only talking to you. *(Milliken, p 135)*

3.

C. Teamwork is the key to good office harmony. When someone needs your help, teamwork dictates that you help them. By telling Janie's doctor she is behind, you may be creating friction between yourself and Janie. *(Hurlbut, p 61)*

4.

C. When you check a blood pressure that seems unusual, the next step is to check the patient's chart to see if it is markedly different from the last time. If it is, and you think your reading is

not correct, check that the cuff is calibrated correctly, check that the cuff was completely deflated, check that you are using a correctly sized cuff, and check B/P in the other arm. If it is still unusual, you can get your superior to check. Remember to always document your findings. *(self)*

5.

B. The correct way to indicate an error is to mark through it once and date and initial it. Never try to cover up an error in any way, because it is a legal document, which might look suspicious if errors are hidden. *(Kinn, p 219)*

6.

C. Information discovered in the office environment is confidential and should be treated as such. You will only comment on Mary's pregnancy if she comments first. *(Milliken, p 266)*

7.

B. To answer in any way that lets this person know that the doctor IS in fact being sued is a breach of confidentiality. Your best answer is to politely and noncommittally say that any information concerning whether or not your doctor is being sued would be confidential. *(Milliken, p 286)*

8.

C. You can recertify with AAMA after becoming a certified medical assistant (CMA) by retaking the exam or obtaining 60 continuing education units (CEUs) every 5 years. *(Lindh, p 8)*

9.

C. Loyalty to your practice includes confidentiality about what goes on in your office. Everyone does have different views so it is best not to prejudice someone by giving your view. *(Milliken, p 286)*

10.

D. However festive you want to be, in a professional environment, it is still best to be conservative. Perfume of any kind is not used in a medical setting, because many people are allergic. Underwear showing through your uniform is completely nonprofessional. Painted nails, especially artificial ones, may often harbor germs in the chipped areas. *(Kinn, p 118)*

4 Patient Communication

contents

I. BEHAVIORAL INFLUENCES

A. *Maslow's hierarchy of needs:* one must fulfill one's own needs in order to relate to others, and use one's talents to the fullest
   1. Physiological (thirst, hunger, sleep, sex)
   2. Safety
   3. Love and belonging
   4. Self-worth and esteem
   5. Self-actualization (reaching one's potential)
   6. Transcendence (spiritualism)

B. *Elizabeth Kubler-Ross:* death and dying stages
   1. Denial (not me!)
   2. Anger (why me?)
   3. Bargaining
   4. Depression
   5. Acceptance

C. *"Know thyself":* one must have self-knowledge to understand others
   1. Knowledge of own values
   2. Understanding of cultural differences
   3. Understanding of patients' perceptions of illness
      a. Loss of job due to illness may cause anxiety and anger
      b. Loss of independence due to illness may cause depression
   4. Defense mechanisms
      a. **Repression:** pushing unpleasant thoughts into unconsciousness
      b. **Displacement:** transferring of one's own feelings to another
      c. **Projection:** blaming another for one's own faults
      d. **Rationalization:** justification of behavior by giving acceptable reasons for behavior rather than the real reason
      e. **Withdrawal:** retreat from the painful situation
   5. **Malingering:** pretending to be ill to avoid unpleasant problems

II. EFFECTIVE TECHNIQUES OF COMMUNICATION
Sender-receiver feedback is essential!

A. Silent periods so that patient can voice feelings

B. Good listening skills
   1. Practice of active, involved listening
   2. Facial expressions to show acknowledgment of message heard
   3. Leaning of body toward person shows interest
   4. Head nodding encourages the speaker to continue

C. *Open-ended questions:* "Tell me about your pain," instead of "Does it hurt here?"

D. *No false reassurances:* "We'll do the best we can," not "Everything will be fine."

E. *Empathy:* putting oneself in another person's place to realize the other person's feelings

F. *Good eye contact*

G. *Repetition:* repeating what is said to be sure it was understood correctly (especially doctor's orders, phone numbers, order numbers, lab reports)

H. *Clarification and feedback ("Do you mean...")*

I. *Special cases:* all persons have self-worth; all persons are unique; treat all without judging
   1. **Deaf and elderly:** speak face to face in case they read lips; treat them as adults, have patience, and allow independent decision making
   2. **Children:** give directions in terms they can understand
   3. **Angry patients:** speak softly, take them to a private area, try to calm them down, and get to the bottom of the problem
   4. **Anxious patients:** give simple directions; give written directions; recognize and accept anxiety; listen to and acknowledge fears
   5. **Cultural differences:** may have to find alternative treatment if patient will not comply for cultural or religious reasons
   6. **Teenagers:** allow privacy; treat as adults
   7. **Dying patients:** acknowledge grief; listen to fears; give no false reassurances
   8. **Blind:** speak in a normal tone of voice; have arm available and let them know it's there for guidance if needed
   9. **Illiterate:** read all consent forms; go over all written information

III. NONEFFECTIVE COMMUNICATION

A. *Criticism and lecturing:* "You don't help your situation when you don't take your medicine."

B. *Preaching:* "Don't you know smoking is wrong?"

C. *False reassurances:* "Everything will be fine."

D. *Changing the subject:* "It sure is sunny today."

E. *Put-downs:* "You shouldn't be afraid of the doctor."

F. *Closed questions (questions answered by one word such as "yes" or "no"):* "Are you hurting?"

key concepts

• Isn't it odd that people raise their voices when speaking to the blind?

G. *Stereotyping or prejudices:* **Most people can sense your inner feelings. This may interfere with communication and understanding. Work at being nonjudgmental.**

IV. BODY LANGUAGE

A. *Facial expression:* **nonverbal behavior**
   1. **Congruence:** verbal and nonverbal message should be the same for good communication
   2. **Expressions should be nonjudgmental**
   3. **Eye contact should be maintained to show interest**

B. *Touch:* **can show sensitivity as long as receiver is accepting of touch**

C. **Posture**
   1. **Standing straight:** promotes the idea of self-assurance
   2. **Slumped posture:** promotes the idea of depression, or lack of confidence
   3. **Arms crossed:** promotes an opinionated, unapproachable image

D. **Movements**
   1. **Drumming of the fingers:** boredom, impatience
   2. **Scratching the head:** puzzlement, confusion
   3. **Tapping the foot:** impatience

E. **Personal space**
   1. **Shorter distances between people indicate more intimate communication**

F. *Clothing and appearance:* **send messages of professionalism or slovenliness**
   1. **Professional:** crisp, clean white uniform
   2. **Nonprofessional:** shirttail out, hair uncombed, runs in hose, unkempt

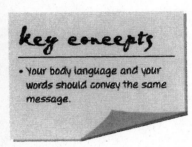

key concepts

• Your body language and your words should convey the same message.

V. TELEPHONE COMMUNICATION

A. **First impression of the office; therefore, answer pleasantly**
   1. Identity of office and of self (and caller)

B. **Hold the receiver close to mouth**

C. **Types of calls received**
   1. **Appointments**
   2. **Prescriptions**
   3. **Test results**

4. **Emergencies:** may need to triage (prioritize according to most severe)
   a. High fevers
   b. Acute illnesses
   c. Medication allergies (possible anaphylaxis)
   d. Dehydration
5. **Doctor's calls or referrals**
   a. Necessity to put through to the doctor right away, but try to have patient's chart in doctor's hand before connecting doctor to caller
6. **Messages**
   a. All messages should be just as readable as any other documentation
   b. Include time of message, sender, receiver, and action to be taken

review questions

DIRECTIONS (Questions 1 through 10): Each of the numbered items or incomplete statements in this section is followed by answers or by completions of the statement. Select the ONE lettered answer or completion that is BEST in each case.

1. Tips for assisting and communicating with a blind patient include
   A. speaking in a voice that is a little louder than usual
   B. placing your hand at the patient's back to guide them to the exam room
   C. letting them know your arm is available for guidance if they wish to take it
   D. maintaining eye contact even though they cannot see

2. The most appropriate action in response to a terminal patient's request to plan his funeral is to
   A. say, "Let's not talk about that right now."
   B. reassure the patient they will be better
   C. pick up the phone and call the family members
   D. respond, "You would like to plan your funeral?"

3. The most appropriate way to help a new patient feel comfortable is to
   A. address them as "sweetheart" or "hon"
   B. put your arm around them as you guide them to the exam room
   C. introduce yourself and provide information about the first visit
   D. call them by their first name

4. An example of congruence of verbal and nonverbal behavior is
   A. looking at your watch when asking a patient how he feels
   B. rolling your eyes when apologizing to the patient for the doctor's emergency
   C. the patient shouts, "I'm not angry about this bill!"
   D. the patient wipes a tear and states, "I am worried about having surgery."

5. Which patient should be escorted to the exam room first?
   A. a patient who has just received an injection, but returns with complaints of itchy palms and feet
   B. a patient with cancer
   C. a postsurgery patient
   D. an epileptic patient

6. Medical assistants communicate professionalism through
   A. a "know-it-all" attitude
   B. chewing gum for sweet-smelling breath
   C. working through lunch, eating at the front desk
   D. team playing

7. A rule to follow when working with the elderly patient is to
   A. speak directly to them as adults
   B. speak to a family member to save time
   C. speak to them as children since they digress with age
   D. call a family member after the visit to explain the patient's condition

8. Which of the following is nonverbal communication?
   A. saying hello
   B. stating the time of day
   C. shaking the head
   D. apologizing to a co-worker

9. Which of the following is a barrier to communication?
   A. changing the subject
   B. silence
   C. restating what the patient just said
   D. repeating the doctor's orders

10. Identify the positive nonverbal behavior below
    A. drumming the fingers
    B. nodding the head
    C. crossing the arms
    D. crossing your leg away from the patient

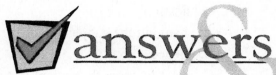

answers & rationales

1.

C. While every person is an individual, most people would rather you offer your arm and let them know it is there if they wish to take it rather than guiding them. By giving them a choice you are fostering independence. You do not speak louder for they are blind not deaf. *(Fremgen, p 522)*

2.

D. Changing the subject, reassuring terminal patients that they will get better, or not talking about dying is unhealthy communication. Terminal patients need to settle their affairs before dying, and planning for the days to come may give them some sense of satisfaction and control. Reflecting what they say gives them a chance to get things off of their minds. *(Milliken, pp 364, 379)*

3.

C. Undue familiarity may make patients more ill at ease. Some people have a certain area around them that is reserved for close relations. This is called their intimate space. By introducing yourself and giving information about what is to be done, you will decrease the patient's anxiety on the first visit. *(Milliken, pp 254–64)*

4.

D. Congruence of verbal and nonverbal behavior is having your actions match your words. If you are talking about happy things, you are smiling. Looking at your watch suggests you have no time for conversation. Rolling your eyes and shouting suggest you are displeased. *(Milliken, p 318)*

5.

A. Of these patients, the most critical one to escort to the back is the one with itchy palms and soles. They may be having a severe allergic reaction called anaphylaxis. *(Lindh, p 207)*

6.

D. Team playing promotes professionalism. Being a know-it-all, chewing gum, or eating at the receptionist desk when greeting patients do not. *(Milliken, p 318)*

7.

A. Although calling a member of the family to further explain an elderly patient's condition is good if you have the patient's permission to release confidential information, the best answer is to speak directly to the patient as an adult. The very elderly may sometimes act childish if they have a degenerative brain disease, but you still treat them with respect and dignity. *(Fremgen, p 522)*

8.

C. All of the answers are verbal responses except shaking the head, which is nonverbal. *(Milliken, p 299)*

9.

A. Silence, repeating, and restating are all good communication tactics, while changing the subject is a barrier to good communication. *(Milliken, p 257)*

10.

B. While nonverbal behavior does not always send the message you might interpret, it may still send out negative messages. Drumming the fingers may send an impatient message; crossing the arms may close communication or indicate you are upset; and crossing the leg away from someone may indicate your wish not to participate in conversation. Nodding the head seems to indicate you are listening and responding. *(Milliken, p 299)*

CHAPTER

5 Medical Law

contents

I. LEGAL TERMS

A. *Ethics:* relating to a set of moral values or actions

B. *Respondeat superior ("Let the master answer"):* doctrine that states that the employer is responsible for the actions of an employee

C. *Medical practice acts:* state statutes that define the practice of medicine

D. *Standard of care:* measurement requiring a doctor to use the ordinary, reasonable skill, experience, and knowledge used by other reputable physicians under the same or similar circumstances in caring for patients

E. *Contract:* agreement between two or more competent persons upon consideration or payment to do or not to do a specific legal activity. The parties must be of legal age or emancipated. There must be acceptance of the contract and something of value exchanged.

F. *Tort:* wrongful act of one person against another that causes harm to person or property

G. *Agent:* a person representing or acting for another

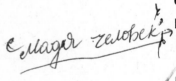

H. *Arbitration:* procedure by which an impartial person, selected by the parties involved, resolves a dispute at a hearing

I. *Emancipated minor:* person under the age of 18 years who is financially independent

J. *False imprisonment:* detention against a person's will

K. Invasion of privacy: disclosure of a person's private affairs without prior consent

L. *Malpractice:* professional misconduct; lack of skill; wrongful practice that causes injury to the patient

M. *Negligence:* not doing an act that a prudent person would do, resulting in injury

N. *Four Ds of negligence:* duty, derelict, direct cause, damages

O. *Res ipsa loquitur ("the thing speaks for itself"):* doctrine where there is an inference of negligence due to the attendant circumstances, e.g., medical malpractice evidenced by a pair of scissors sewn up in a patient

P. *Privileged communication:* that which cannot be made public, as that which arises from the doctor-patient relationship

Q. *Statute of limitations:* specific period of time in which a lawsuit can be filed or initiated

R. *Subpoena duces tecum:* an order to provide records or documents to the court

S. *Locum tenens:* substitute or representative

T. *Liability:* obligation by law to pay or make amends for an act

U. *Scope of practice:* legal bounds within which a person practices her/his profession

V. *Quid pro quo:* the giving of something in return for something else

II. MALPRACTICE PREVENTION

A. Kindness to patients maintained: sincere caring for patients (generally, patients hate to sue people who have been sincerely kind and caring toward them)

B. Performance within the scope of practice

C. Compliance with state laws

D. Learned knowledge of safe and aseptic practice used

E. Documentation of all patient visits, calls and correspondence, missed appointments, and prescriptions authorized by telephone to the pharmacist

F. No telephone advice given

G. Patient data such as lab reports seen and initialed by doctor prior to filing

H. Confidentiality practiced

I. Cures never guaranteed

J. Explanations of appointment delays given along with apologies

K. Estimates of fees given with explanations that they are just estimates

L. Informed consents secured when needed along with documentation of the discussion held

M. Doctor informed of patient complaints

N. Documentation kept of discharge or release of patients and certified letter sent when withdrawing from a case

key concepts

MALPRACTICE BREACH OF DUTY:
- Malfeasance—the care performed by the doctor is illegal
- Misfeasance—not performing legal care correctly
- Nonfeasance—not performing care that should have been given

III. PHYSICIAN REGULATIONS

A. *Controlled Substances Act:* **regulates dispensing of scheduled drugs**

   1. **Registration with the DEA (Drug Enforcement Agency):** renewal every three years

   2. **Record keeping:** include patient given drug, dosage, route, date given, and reason given; records kept two years

   3. **Inventory:** on date of registration and every two years following date of initial inventory

   4. **Drug schedules**

     a. **I:** highest potential for abuse; not legalized (marijuana)

     b. **II:** high abuse potential, but accepted medically; must use special DEA form in triplicate (quaalude, codeine, morphine, opium derivatives, stimulants, amphetamines)

     c. **III:** less abuse potential; may become dependent (amphetamine-like substances, narcotic drugs with limited amounts of codeine)

     d. **IV:** lower abuse potential (valium, minor tranquilizers)

     e. **V:** least potential for abuse (lomotil, drugs with limited amounts of narcotics)

   5. Log of controlled drugs with patient name, drug, dosage, and date given

     a. **Patient's chart:** record of controlled drugs given should agree with log

     b. **Wasting of drugs:** log and have witness

B. **Physician licensure requirements**

   1. Legal age

   2. Moral character

   3. Completion of all educational requirements and passing of boards

   4. Renewal

     a. Periodically (usually yearly, with proof of 50 hours of CEUs)

   5. Revocation/suspension

     a. Conviction of crime

     b. Unprofessional conduct

     c. Personal or professional incapacity

C. **Uniform Anatomical Gift Act**

   1. Patient donation of body or parts of body after death for research or transplant

     a. Sound mind and legal age required

     b. No money exchange

     c. Time of death determined by a doctor having no interest in the transplant or research

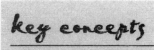

key concepts

FOUR Ds OF NEGLIGENCE:
- Duty to a patient
- Derelict in that duty
- Damages resulting in poor care
- Directly caused by poor care

D. Living will
1. Patients elect not to receive life-sustaining measures if a life-threatening event takes place (must be decided prior to any life-threatening event)
    a. Competency of patient a must
    b. Two witnesses needed

E. *Medical practice acts:* define practices for physicians in each state
1. Doctor must practice within the scope of his/her training and not beyond the limits of his/her state's medical practice acts

F. *Public health duties*
1. Reports to proper authorities
    a. Vital statistics: birth, death, and fetal death
    b. Communicable diseases
    c. Known or suspected abuse
    d. Drug abuse
    e. Criminal acts

G. *Informed consent:* consent for an invasive procedure after the patient is informed of risks, the procedure itself, alternative treatments, and possible results if treatment is not performed. After patient signs an informed consent, it is appropriate to document in the patient's chart that questions were answered to the patient's satisfaction and a discussion of risks, alternative treatments, and so on, was held.

H. *Worker's compensation:* doctor must register with state worker's compensation boards yearly

IV. MEDICAL OFFICE REGULATIONS

A. *Truth-in-Lending Act, Regulation Z:* any bill paid in more than four installments must be written and an indication made as to whether or not interest will be charged

B. *CLIA (Clinical Laboratory Improvement Amendments):* medical office laboratories must follow certain regulations for quality assurance

C. *Hazardous wastes:* must be disposed of according to OSHA (Occupational Safety and Health Act) requirements

D. *OSHA (Occupational Safety and Health Act):* sets standards and regulations for occupational health and safety
1. Hazard plan
2. Exposure plan

3. Waste management
4. Environmental and housekeeping plan
5. Personal protective barriers
6. General and fire safety
7. Training in-house

E. *Taxes:* **federal, state, and local guidelines must be adhered to**
1. All new employees must fill out W-4 forms (employee's withholding allowance certificate)
2. W-2 forms must be given by January 31 (wage and tax statements)
3. **FICA:** Federal Insurance Contributions Act—Social Security taxes (employer and employee contribute)
   a. **OASI:** Old Age and Survivors Insurance
   b. **HI:** hospitalization under Medicare
   c. **DI:** disability insurance
4. **FUTA:** Federal Unemployment Tax Act (employer contributions only)
5. **Gross earnings:** amount actually made
6. **Net earnings:** amount given employee after taxes and other deductions

F. *Release of patient information:* **always need permission and signature of patient to release any medical information**

G. *Sexual harassment:* **Sexual discrimination that is gender-based; job advancement offered in exchange for sexual favors; inappropriate touching**

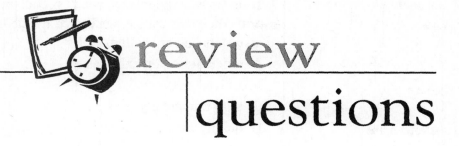

review questions

DIRECTIONS (Questions 1 through 10): Each of the numbered items or incomplete statements in this section is followed by answers or by completions of the statement. Select the ONE lettered answer or completion that is BEST in each case.

---

1. A medical assistant's scope of practice
   A. may vary from state to state
   B. is the same across the nation
   C. is the same as an LPN
   D. allows all certified medical assistants to practice the same

2. A medical assistant can
   A. perform x-rays in all states
   B. never perform x-rays in any state
   C. perform x-rays in most states that do not require licensure to perform x-rays
   D. perform x-rays if they are a certified medical assistant

3. Choose the true statement ending: Medical assisting certification and registration covers all states
   A. therefore, the practice of a medical assistant will not change from state to state
   B. but the practice of a medical assistant may vary from state to state
   C. but you must re-examine when you move to another state
   D. therefore, there is no need to ever reregister or recertify

4. Once tested and licensed, doctors
   A. cannot lose their licenses
   B. have to retest for renewal of their licenses every 6 years
   C. can still lose their licenses for personal incapacity
   D. must have no malpractice suits brought against them to retain their licenses

5. Being sure that a medical assistant performs laboratory procedures within the scope of practice is a job for
   A. OSHA
   B. CLIA
   C. DEA
   D. FICA

6. Fire extinguishers in an office may be regulated by
   A. COLA
   B. OSHA
   C. FEMA
   D. FDA

7. To perform minor surgery on a patient but charge for major surgery would be
   A. assault
   B. battery
   C. fraud
   D. disclaimer

8. Reportable incidences do not include
   A. birth of a baby
   B. death of a patient
   C. child abuse
   D. a case of Parkinson's disease

9. Examples of controlled substances are
   A. narcotics only
   B. nonnarcotics only
   C. narcotics and some nonnarcotics
   D. Schedule VII drugs

10. Tests such as pregnancy, occult blood, and urine dipsticks can be performed by medical assistants and are called
    A. moderate-complexity tests
    B. waived tests
    C. high-complexity tests
    D. quality assurance tests

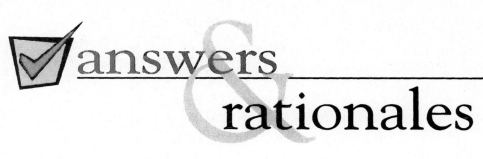

answers & rationales

1.

A. Medical practice acts vary from state to state. Most states do not even have medical practice acts for medical assistants. Because the scope of practice for other occupations changes from state to state, it affects the scope of practice for medical assistants. For instance, in some states, one must be licensed to perform x-rays; therefore, medical assistants could not perform x-rays. Other states have unlicensed personnel performing simple x-rays. *(Lindh, p 10; Fremgen, pp 7–12)*

2.

C. see question #1

3.

B. see question #1

4.

C. Doctors can lose their license for personal incapacity. *(Fremgen, pp 27–30)*

5.

B. CLIA (Clinical Laboratory Improvement Amendments) spells out which tests in a laboratory are routine and which ones require more in-depth education. *(Kinn, p 837)*

6.

B. OSHA (Occupational Safety and Health Administration) regulates fire extinguishers in a doctor's office. Once in place, OSHA requires personnel to be trained on how to use them, or if there are no fire extinguishers, there must be a fixed evacuation plan. *(Kinn, p 73, pp 419–21)*

7.

C. Fraud is being deceitful. To do one procedure and charge for another is deceitful practice. Assault is threat of bodily harm, and battery is doing bodily harm. A disclaimer is stating lack of responsibility for something that may happen. *(Fremgen, p 77)*

8.

D. Parkinson's disease is not communicable so it is not a reportable illness. Births, deaths, and child abuse are all reportable actions that are the physician's public duty to report. Reportable diseases may vary from state to state but are usually communicable. *(Kinn, p 76)*

9.

C. Controlled substances by the DEA are substances that may be addicting. They may be narcotics or nonnarcotic. *(DEA; Kinn, p 75)*

10.

B. Waived tests are low-complexity tests and can be performed by the medical assistant. Occult blood on feces, routine urine dipsticks, and visual color comparison pregnancy tests are all waived tests. *(Kinn, p 837)*

CHAPTER

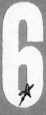

Written Communication

contents

I. FORMATS

Standard stationery in a professional medical office is usually 16- to 24-pound weight and 8½ by 11 inches. Elite type is the best choice for professional correspondence.

A. Letters

1. **Full block:** date, inside address, salutation, body, complimentary closing, typed signature, and initials are flush left margin
   a. No tabs needed

key concepts

• Using the full block format is the fastest because there are no tabs for indentations.

Tony Moore, M.D.
100 Drivers Lane
Winterville, NC 28590

August 4, 1994

Jarrett Tucker, M.D.
Greenville Boulevard
Hills Point, NC 48567

Dear Doctor Tucker:

I appreciate your referring Jeff Stallings. He was seen in our office today. My examination revealed nothing remarkable.

I am requesting a CAT scan of the brain. His appointment is 8-16-94. He will return on 8-20-94 to discuss the scan.

Sincerely yours,

Tony Moore, M.D.

aph

FIGURE 6–1 Full block format.

2. **Modified block:** date, complimentary closing, and typed signature a little to the right of center, with all three lining up
   a. Professional-looking with most letterheads
3. **Modified block with indented paragraphs:** date, complimentary closing, and typed signature a little to the right of center, all three lining up; each paragraph usually indented five spaces
   a. Least popular, probably because of the time it takes to tabulate
4. **General rules**
   a. **Months:** spelled out
   b. **Doctors:** use Joe Barnes, M.D. instead of Dr. Joe Barnes
   c. **Salutation:** followed by a colon in professional correspondence

Tony Moore, M.D.
100 Drivers Lane
Winterville, NC 28590

August 4, 1994

Jarrett Tucker, M.D.
Greenville Boulevard
Hills Point, NC 48567

Dear Doctor Tucker:

Jeff Stallings

I appreciate your referring Jeff Stallings. He was seen in our office today. My examination revealed nothing remarkable.

I am requesting a CAT scan of the brain. His appointment is 8-16-94. He will return on 8-20-94 to discuss the scan.

Sincerely yours,

Tony Moore, M.D.

aph

FIGURE 6–2   Modified block format.

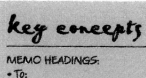

key concepts

PARTS OF A PROFESSIONAL LETTER:
• Date
• Inside address
• Salutation
• Subject line (optional)
• Body of letter
• Complimentary closing
• Signature
• Reference initials

Tony Moore, M.D.
100 Drivers Lane
Winterville, NC 28590

August 4, 1994

Jarrett Tucker, M.D.
Greenville Boulevard
Hills Point, NC 48567

Dear Doctor Tucker:

        I appreciate your referring Jeff Stallings. He was seen in our office today. My examination revealed nothing remarkable.

        I am requesting a CAT scan of the brain. His appointment is 8-16-94. He will return on 8-20-94 to discuss the scan.

Sincerely yours,

Tony Moore, M.D.

aph

FIGURE 6–3   Modified block with indented paragraphs.

key concepts

MEMO HEADINGS:
• To:
• From:
• Date:
• Subject:

    d. Double spacing between paragraphs

    e. First word only of the closing is capitalized (Yours truly)

    f. **Elite:** 12 characters per inch (usual professional type)

    g. **Pica:** 10 characters per inch (good for reports and speeches)

    h. Second pages

      • Name of addressee typed on seventh line

      • Page number

      • Date

      • Body of letter typed on tenth line

B. Memos

1. Margin: flush left and double spaced; four lines of headings (names, date, and subject information) should line up on tabulation at tenth space as shown next:

MEMORANDUM

MEMO TO: Virginia Perkins, Manager

FROM: Jenny Hemby

DATE: January 9, 2001

SUBJECT: Annual Evaluations

(Leave two blank lines before the body of MEMORANDUM, and single-space body)

2. No paragraph indention

3. 2-inch top margin for a full sheet; 1-inch top margin for a half sheet

C. Reports

1. Add ½ inch to the left margin (or margin and tab stops three spaces to the right), if bound

2. Paragraphs indented five spaces

3. Double space

4. First page, 2-inch top margin; other pages, 1-inch top margin

5. Bottom margin: 1 inch

D. Tables

1. All-cap single-spaced title

2. Body is centered horizontally

3. Word columns align left; number columns align right

4. Decimals aligned

E. Manuscripts

1. Format is the same as that of bound reports

II. EDITING

A. *Watermark:* **a mark seen through bond paper when held up to the light**
1. **Correct side of bonded paper:** type on paper in same direction as watermark can be read

B. *Erasable bond:* **type on the correct side (erasable side)**

C. Proofreader's Marks

⌃	Insert comma	v̇	Insert apostrophe
v̇ v̇	Insert quotation marks	⊙	Insert period
⊙	Insert colon	;)	Insert semicolon
?/	Insert question mark	=/	Insert hyphen
⌐	Delete	⌒	Close up
¶	Paragraph	∽	Transpose
#	Insert space	⊏	Move left
⊐	Move right	⑤℗	Spell out
≡	Capitals	lc	Lower case

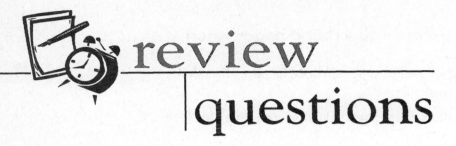
review questions

DIRECTIONS (Questions 1 through 10): Each of the numbered items or incomplete statements in this section is followed by answers or by completions of the statement. Select the ONE lettered answer or completion that is BEST in each case.

1. A professional letter that can be finished in less time because there are no tabs is formatted in
   A. full block
   B. modified block
   C. modified block with indentations
   D. a casual style-flush left

2. You would never write one of the following phrases in professional correspondence:
   A. Dear Doctor Hemby:
   B. Yours truly, Gene Hemby, M.D.
   C. Gene Hemby, M.D. (inside address)
   D. Yours Truly, Gene Hemby, M.D.

3. Choose the rule that is incorrect
   A. double-space between paragraphs in letters
   B. double-space between each memo heading
   C. single-space speeches
   D. single-space body of memo

4. A written message should include
   A. date and time of message
   B. the message taker's name or initials
   C. action to be taken on the message
   D. all of the above

In questions 5–10, choose the correctly written communication.

5.
   A. He were there yesterday.
   B. She come in to have her blood pressure checked.
   C. He was pass the normal lab values.
   D. She is a pleasant patient.

6.
   A. A child's blood pressure cup was used.
   B. She has an optomologist consult.
   C. I appreciate your referring Mrs. Jones.
   D. We saw many patience yesterday.

7.
   A. We have many magazine prescriptions in the waiting area.
   B. The patient was seen by their appointment times.
   C. Mrs. Jones was given Mrs. Smith's appointment.
   D. I hardly reconized Mrs. Jones.

8.
   A. The optometrist performed the surgery.
   B. The instrument is sterile.
   C. She was worried about her sugery.
   D. He preformed cardiopulmonary resuscitation.

9.
   A. The lab report is her's.
   B. The qrs complex is normal.
   C. The drug is an Analgesic.
   D. The diagnosis is Hodgkin's disease.

10.
   A. He was given an injection, a prescription and a nebulizer.
   B. Before the beginning of the procedure he was told to move as little as possible.
   C. She said according to her daughter that she did not take her medicine.
   D. She is a well-nourished female.

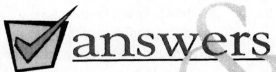

answers & rationales

1.

A. Full block is often used for professional correspondence. There are no tabs or indentions so it takes less time to key in. Any casual style would not be used in professional correspondence. *(Kinn, p 146)*

2.

D. All are correct except "Yours Truly." In this complimentary closing the "t" in truly would NOT be capitalized. *(Kinn, p 149)*

3.

C. All rules are correct except c. Speeches would be double-spaced to be more easily read. *(Fordney)*

4.

D. A written message should include the date and time of the message, the message itself, who the message is for, the action to be taken on the message, who the message is from, and who took the message in case there are any questions. If the call is to be returned, you must also get the telephone number, and a convenient time to call back. *(Fordney)*

5.

D. To correct the other answers, you would change were to was in a, change come to came in b, and change pass to past in c. *(Fordney)*

6.

C. To correct the others, you would change cup to cuff in a, change optomologist to ophthalmology, and in d, change patience to patients. *(Fordney)*

7.

C. To correct the others, you would change prescriptions to subscriptions, change patient was seen to patients were seen, and in d, reconized should be spelled recognized. *(Fordney)*

8.

B. Choice a should read the ophthalmologist because optometrists do not perform surgery. In c, sugery should be spelled surgery, and in d, preformed should be spelled performed. *(Fordney)*

9.

D. In a, her's should be hers, qrs should be QRS in b, and in c, Analgesic should be analgesic. *(Fordney)*

10.

D. A comma should be placed after prescription in a, a comma should be placed after procedure in b, and according to her daughter should be set off by commas in c. *(Fordney)*

7 Office Equipment

I. GENERAL OFFICE MACHINES

A. Calculator/adding machine

1. **Features:** digital display and tape for permanent record
2. **Use:** billing, bank deposits, daily reports, and financial transactions

B. Copy machine

1. **Features:** different-sized papers, contrast, and settings for number of copies, size reduction, size increase, and collation
2. **Use:** copying instruction sheets, correspondence for patient files, reports, and bills

C. Check writer

1. **Features:** settings for date, name of payee, and amount of check
2. **Use:** for writing checks that cannot be altered

D. Postage meter and scales

1. **Features:** prints postage on the envelope or on tabs to put on the envelope
2. **Use:** scales weigh mail to obtain accurate postage and meters dispense exact postage; letters do not have to be canceled or postmarked (saving time)

E. Intercom, voice mail, and electronic mail

1. **Features:** can be part of a telephone system
   a. **Intercom:** can transfer calls or speak within the office without yelling
   b. **Voice mail:** recording gives prompts for person calling to touch certain numbers and then record a message
   c. **E-mail:** mail sent electronically from computer to computer
2. **Use:** for paging parties to the phone or speaking from one room to the next; interoffice oral communication

F. Beeper

1. **Features:** compact and mobile; lets person know what number to call
2. **Use:** can be worn anywhere, so office staff can be in touch with the person wearing the beeper at all times

G. Fax (facsimile) machine

1. **Features:** quick means of sending and receiving information on paper through use of telecommunications
2. **Use:** can quickly send copies of lab reports, physical findings, and so on, from one place to another via telecommunications
   a. Confidentiality must still be practiced with fax machines

H. Dictation machines

1. **Features:** speed up, slow down, replay, foot pedals, and earphones

---

key concepts

• Any time you are about to purchase a new office machine, obtain input from employees as to features needed on that machine. Then call several different companies to come and demonstrate their machine prior to purchase.

2. **Use:** listen to doctor's recorded tapes for transcribing and placement in charts

I. Answering machines

1. **Features:** settings for number of rings before pickup, can record and change own message, call back for messages, skip, replay, rewind, and fast forward
2. **Use**
   a. Answers phone and records message of caller
   b. Screens incoming calls prior to answering

II. COMPUTERS

A. Terminology

1. **Disk drive:** unit in which a diskette or CD is inserted to obtain information from or to put information onto a diskette or CD
   a. Zip drive/Zip disk—used to store excessive information; Zip disks hold more than regular disks
2. **Screen or monitor:** unit that displays processed information
3. **Function keys:** keys for performing certain tasks (as in centering) and help keys (help-key: usually F1 but can vary depending on the software package)
4. **Backup:** copies of existing data are available so that information will not be lost
5. **Cursor:** a marker that shows where the next character will be typed or the next function will take place
6. **Fonts:** character types
7. **Hard copy:** the printout on paper of information from the screen
8. **Initialize or format:** prepare a diskette for information storage
9. **Menu:** display of functions from which to choose
10. **Peripheral:** anything added to or plugged into the computer
11. **Software:** various programs that direct the computer to do certain functions
12. **Scrolling:** moving up or down through information
13. **Modem:** connects computer to other computers for communication via telephone lines
    a. Dictation to another computer by phone
    b. Electronic claims processing
    c. Voice mail
14. **CPU:** central processing unit
15. **Hardware:** physical equipment (CPU, printer, keyboard, and monitor)
16. **Password:** any alphanumeric series used as a way to get into a secured menu (e.g., payroll)
17. **Tutorial:** a program that teaches use of the software

18. **Commands:** certain words and symbols in a form and sequence to get the computer to do certain tasks (e.g., the command "Format a:" will format a disk)

B. Uses

1. Word processing
   a. Patient data input
   b. Correspondence
   c. Reports
   d. Patient educational materials
2. Billing and financial transactions (can process superbills for each patient daily with procedures and diagnoses and their CPT, ICD-9 CM, and HCPCS codes)
3. Insurance processing
   a. Electronic claims processing by telecommunication
4. Payroll
5. Year-end reports
6. Aging accounts
7. Activity analysis
8. Appointment scheduling
9. Accounts receivable reports (total amount all patients owe)
10. End-of-month statements
11. Database of all patients

C. Maintenance

1. Instruction booklets to be read and followed
2. Maintenance contracts and service agreements for designated price per month or year
3. Computer diskettes
   a. Disk varieties
      - Size of diskettes: $5\frac{1}{4}$, $3\frac{1}{2}$, and 8 inches
      - Density of disketttes: DD (double density), HD (high density), and SD (single density)
      - Types of diskettes: floppy, floppy with hard case, CD, Zip
   b. Maintenance
      - No temperature extremes
      - Avoidance of dust, smoke, food, drink, and magnetic fields
      - Any label must be written on before attaching to the diskette, or written with a soft-tip pen
      - Diskette must never be forced into the drive

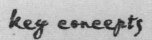

key concepts

- When purchasing office equipment, always inquire about maintenance contracts, cost of parts, service and support from company, and warranties.

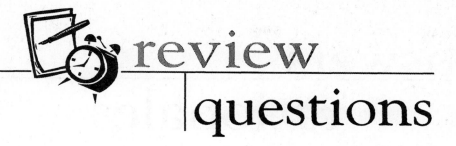

review questions

DIRECTIONS In questions 1–4, choose the office machine you would use for the following actions.

1. To leave a recorded message
   A. fax machine
   B. voice mail
   C. dictation machine
   D. CPU

2. To let the doctor know he is needed at the office when he is on rounds
   A. intercom
   B. beeper
   C. voice mail
   D. fax

3. To do end-of-month reports
   A. dictation machine
   B. Zip drive
   C. computer
   D. e-mail

4. To send a lab report copy to the hospital
   A. answering machine
   B. fax machine
   C. beeper
   D. voice mail

DIRECTIONS (Questions 5 through 10): Each of the numbered items or incomplete statements in this section is followed by answers or by completions of the statement. Select the ONE lettered answer or completion that is BEST in each case.

5. To begin recording information on a disk, you would first have to
   A. format it
   B. place it in the Zip drive
   C. press F1
   D. change the font

6. To find information not shown at the bottom of the computer monitor, you would have to
   A. move the cursor up
   B. scroll down
   C. perform a backup
   D. use a modem

7. To find out more about your new software, you could run a
   A. tutorial
   B. modem
   C. Zip drive
   D. format command

8. To type letters on a computer, you would use
   A. spreadsheet software
   B. tutorial software
   C. memo wizard
   D. data-processing software

9. To name and save a file, you would use
   A. "save"
   B. "help"
   C. "save as"
   D. "copy"

10. Most professional correspondence will be in
    A. 6–8 font
    B. 10–12 font
    C. 16–18 font
    D. 24–46 font

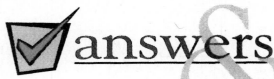
answers & rationales

1.

B. A recorded message can be left on voice mail.
(Fremgen, pp 181–82; self)

2.

B. When the doctor is away from the office and needs to be contacted, you will leave the number to call on his beeper. *(Fremgen, pp 181–82; self)*

3.

C. End-of-the-month reports will be performed on the computer. *(Fremgen, pp 181–82; self)*

4.

B. The fax machine copies a document, and another copy will be reproduced wherever you send it. *(Fremgen, pp 181–82; self)*

5.

A. A disk must be formatted before any information can be recorded onto it. *(Fremgen, pp 181–82; self)*

6.

B. When you move down through information on the computer screen, it is called scrolling down. *(Fremgen, pp 181–82; self)*

7.

A. Many software packages have a tutorial included in the software so that when you run the tutorial, you can learn about the software. *(Fremgen, pp 181–82; self)*

8.

D. Data-processing software must be used to type professional letters on a computer. *(Fremgen, pp 181–82; self)*

9.

C. To name and save a file for the first time you would use "save as." You can also change the name of a file by using "save as." *(Fremgen, pp 181–82; self)*

10.

B. Professional correspondence is usually in the #10–12 font (Times New Roman). *(Fremgen, pp 181–82; self)*

8 Medical Records

I. MAINTENANCE

A. Supplies

1. **Tabs:** for color coding names, dates, insurance, and so on
   a. Color coding—makes it easy to spot misfiled charts.
   b. Year tabs—help spot the last year patient was seen
2. **Folders:** condition (repair) folders when necessary
3. **Outguides and outfolders:** may tell where a chart is or give a place to put papers until the chart is replaced

B. *Shingling:* placing reports one over the other with bottom tab showing for organization

C. Filing systems

1. **Geographic:** file by area or location, then in alphabetical or numerical sequence
2. **Chronologic:** file by date
   a. **Tickler file:** a reminder system set up like a calendar by dates
3. **Alphabetic:** file by ABC order, usually last name (surname) first
   Example: Langston, Betty
   a. "Nothing before something"
      Example: Smith is filed before Smithson
   b. "Last the same, try first name"
      Example: Langston, Blake before Langston, Jim
   c. When THE is part of a business name, consider it the last indexing unit
      Example: The Dime Store: Unit 1 = Dime, Unit 2 = Store, Unit 3 = The
   d. Titles are not considered
      Example: Professor John Smith and Sam Smith
      Smith, John (Professor) first, then Smith, Sam
   e. Hyphenated names are considered one unit
      Example: Jones-Johnson, John before Jonesrude, John
4. **Numeric:** file by a numbering system, usually the smallest number to the largest disregarding any zeros in front of a number
   Example: 0012 before 014
   a. Cross-reference needed to be able to look up a patient's name alphabetically to find their chart number
   b. Terminal digit: in numbers such as 22-33-45, use the last two digits to sort files first, then the middle digits, then the first digits
      Example: 22-33-45 before 22-35-45
5. **Subject:** file by heading or subject area
   a. Subject list needed for ease in filing

key concepts

• A patient must sign a form to release his/her records before the medical office can file insurance or transfer records to another office.

D. Filing steps

1. **Inspection and release:** checking to see if all action on information is completed before filing
   Example: doctor looks at lab report and initials it before it can be filed
2. **Indexing:** deciding under which subject the information should be filed
3. **Coding:** marking to show under which subject the information is to be filed
4. **Sorting:** organizing material to be filed before actually filing it
5. **Storing:** locating the proper place for filing and storing the information

II. STORAGE AND EQUIPMENT

A. *File cabinets:* Vertical, lateral, drawer, automatic, and shelf

B. *Card index files*

C. *Microfilm and diskettes*

D. *Inactive files:* files of patients who have not been seen in a specified period of time or of patients who have died; may be stored in special boxes in controlled storage
   1. Purging—periodically removing inactive files according to oldest year tabs to make room for new charts

E. *Closed files:* files of patients who will never return; deceased patients.

III. CONFIDENTIALITY

A. Files are not released without patient authorization
   1. Release of records form must be signed by the patient

B. Numerical filing is more confidential than alphabetical filing because a cross-reference is required

C. Electronic information sent by fax or computer is treated with the same rules of confidentiality

IV. FORMAT

A. POMR: problem-oriented medical record
   1. Organization by patient's problems instead of traditional source-oriented record (information sorted according to who generates it, such as nurses' notes, doctors' notes, or medical assistants' notes)

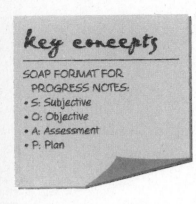

key concepts

SOAP FORMAT FOR
  PROGRESS NOTES:
• S: Subjective
• O: Objective
• A: Assessment
• P: Plan

2. **Database:** patient information
3. **Problems:** any problems needing management will be in SOAP notes or progress notes form; always dated
   a. S = subjective: what patient tells office staff
      Example: "My foot hurts"
   b. O = objective findings: what health care worker (doctor, medical assistant, etc.) finds upon examination
      Example: v/s = T 101 P 72 R 14 B/P 120/90, x-ray—normal
   c. A = assessment: same as Dx (diagnosis)
      Example: A: Arthritis
      Example: A: R/O Arthritis
      Example: A: Arthritis vs. Bursitis
   d. P = plan
      Example: P: ii Getwell tabs TID, Re-check 1 wk.
      Example: P: Chest x-ray, PA and Lat STAT, F/U 1 week

B. Corrections
1. No erasing or whiting out; chart is written in black ink, so mark through once, initial, date, and make corrections above or beside. Some may choose to also write "corr" beside errors.

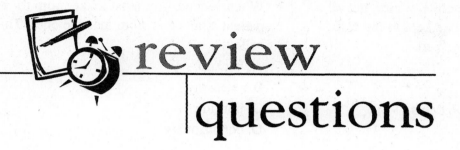

review questions

DIRECTIONS (Questions 1 through 10): Each of the numbered items or incomplete statements in this section is followed by answers or by completions of the statement. Select the ONE lettered answer or completion that is BEST in each case.

---

1. When using the SOAP format for progress notes,
   A. S means source
   B. O means orders
   C. A means assessment
   D. P means prognosis

2. In source-oriented progress notes, a heading that would not be used is
   A. doctor's notes
   B. nurse's notes
   C. lab
   D. objective

3. Choose the sequence in correct alphabetical order.
   A. Smith, Joan   Perkins, Al
      Staton, Sue   Morgan, Jamie
   B. Ness, Bill   Orville, Reid
      Ross, Tim   Mann, Seth
   C. Best, Cal   Fulton, Beth
      High, Joe   Smith, Don
   D. Ross, Al   Russell, Jo
      Ryan, Gil   Pollock, Bea

4. Choose the sequence in correct alphabetical order.
   A. Small, Jack   Smith, Jo
      Smut, Dee   Packard, Sue
   B. Tack, Elaine   Teal, Bo
      Tillman, Gigi   Smyth, Fran

   C. Denis, Mark   Dennis, Sam
      Dennisy, Tom   Dancy, Ned
   D. Gibbs, Mark   Gibbs, Olive
      Gibbs, Oliver   Gibs, Sue

5. Choose the correct terminal digit sequence.
   A. 11-09-11   11-10-12
      12-10-12   12-14-13
   B. 11-22-44   11-22-45
      11-23-45   11-23-33
   C. 11-23-33   11-24-22
      11-45-14   11-46-81
   D. 11-25-46   12-21-47
      11-22-50   13-44-45

6. You have just finished documenting on what you thought was a page of Jane Smith's chart. When you turn the page over to continue, you see that you have documented on Jane Wilson's chart. To correct this error, you will
   A. recopy both sides and place in the correct charts
   B. shred the misdocumented page and go find Jane Smith's chart
   C. line through all of the misdocumented information, write "incorrect chart; rewritten in chart # 11-22-45," and initial and date
   D. obtain a clean sheet and glue it over the misdocumented information

7. Your doctor has three satellite clinics, but all records for those clinics are kept in the main office. They are probably filed
   A. chronologically
   B. geographically
   C. by subject heading "Patients"
   D. in a tickler file

8. When needed, you must repair very active charts. This is called
   A. releasing
   B. conditioning
   C. sorting
   D. coding

9. When needed, you must make room for new patient charts and store inactive ones. This is called
   A. backup
   B. releasing
   C. purging
   D. conditioning

10. Misfiled charts can be spotted easily if you use
    A. terminal digit filing
    B. outguides
    C. date tabs
    D. color-coding tabs

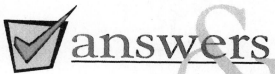

answers & rationales

1.

C. A means Assessment; S means subjective information; O means objective information; P means Plan. *(Kinn, p 214)*

2.

D. Objective would be used in a problem-oriented medical record. *(Lindh, p 251)*

3.

C. Alphabetical order is correct only in c. *(Fremgen, p 238)*

4.

D. The Gibbs and Gibs are in alphabetical order. Since there is more than one Gibbs, you then have to look at the second unit. Mark comes before Olive. Olive comes before Oliver because of the rule that nothing comes before something. *(Lindh, pp 238–39)*

5.

A. In terminal digit filing, you always look at the last set of digits first, then the middle digits, then the first. *(Fremgen, p 238)*

6.

C. The correct and legal way to correct errors is to line through them, initial the error, and date it. *(Kinn, pp 219, 407)*

7.

B. These files will be kept geographically according to the location of the office. If the clinic is in Greenville, you will go to the Greenville satellite charts and then find the correct chart either in alphabetical order or numerical order. *(Hurlbut, p 40)*

8.

B. Repairing charts is called conditioning. *(Hurlbut, p 142)*

9.

C. When purging files, you will remove the inactive files and store them elsewhere to make more room for the active ones. *(Hurlbut, p 144)*

10.

D. When using colored files for the numbers or letters of a chart, the tabs are color coded. When one is misfiled, it stands out easily because it is in a group of like colors and it is the wrong color. *(Fremgen, p 240)*

9 Postal Services

contents

I. CLASSES (BASED ON TYPE, WEIGHT AND DESTINATION)

A. First class: 12 oz or less (standard—less than 1/4" thick)
1. Letters and postcards, sealed or not sealed
2. Green-diamond bordered envelopes
3. Not subject to inspection
4. Standard envelopes
   a. #10, #6¾

B. Second class
1. Newspapers and magazines
2. Bulk mail sent by publishers and others

C. Third class: up to 16 oz
1. Catalogs and photographs
2. Subject to inspection

D. Fourth class: 16 oz or more up to 70 lb (parcel post); maximum dimensions—108 inches, combined length and width
1. Books, films, and manuscripts

E. Combination mailing
1. **Letter and package:** if a letter is inside a package, separate postage must be paid for each, and "letter enclosed" must be written on the package

F. Educational materials
1. Lower rate than fourth class

G. Special services
1. **Special delivery:** same speed of service from city to city, but will be delivered immediately upon arrival to the place of address if served by carriers or within 1 mile of the post office
2. **Express mail:** high-speed delivery; sent by 5 P.M. one day and received by 3 P.M. the next day if delivered, but received by 10 A.M. if picked up by the receiver
3. **Certificate of mailing:** receipt is evidence that item was mailed
4. **Certified mail:** first-class mail with proof of delivery on record for 2 years
5. **Registered mail:** evidence of delivery and added protection; person receiving must sign for mail; any class can be registered; especially useful for items of high value
6. **Insured mail:** third and fourth class should be insured if the value is over $25
7. **Receipt of delivery:** shows date item was received by the person to whom it was sent

8. **Money orders:** safe way of sending money through the mail
9. **Recall of mail:** written request with proper ID, mailer pays expenses
10. **Priority mail:** exceptions to limitations of classes may be sent by "priority" to receive expeditious handling
    a. Rates based on weight and distance
11. **Address correction requested:** use to locate someone who has moved
    a. Post office will forward mail with "address correction requested" and send mailer new address for a fee
12. Biological specimens must have universal precaution hazardous sticker

H. Alternatives to postal service
1. Private services, such as UPS and Federal Express
2. Couriers hired by private concerns, such as laboratories that pick up lab specimens

II. FORMATS

A. OCR read area (automation and Zip codes speed delivery)
1. Automation requires address within a rectangle that is 1 inch from right and left edges, 5/8 inch and 2-3/4 inches up from the bottom
2. USPS bar code sprayed in the bottom right edge for further processing after OCR (optical character reader) reads

B. Sans-serif characters best; script, handwriting, and italics cannot be read by the OCR

C. Maximum contrast best

D. Correct spacing between letters

E. All caps and no punctuation

F. Standard USPS state abbreviations
1. 2 letter abbreviations

G. Zip code on same line as city and state
1. Zip code should be 5+4 digits
   a. +4 indicates city block, large office complex
   b. Nothing below Zip code line
   c. Internet Zip codes: www.usps.gov

H. Software for addressing/labeling
1. Data processing or specialized software
   a. Use "tools" menu and choose envelopes/labeling

III. SORTING INCOMING MAIL

A. Batch by department/doctors

1. Medical assistant will screen and process
2. Open and clip to envelope unless it has inside address, then envelope can be thrown away
3. Stamp date on letter
4. Prioritize—personal mail and checks on top

IV. ELECTRONIC METERS (EXAMPLE: PITNEY BOWES, 1-800-322-8000)

A. Postmarks/cancels mail

B. Use correct date and mail same day

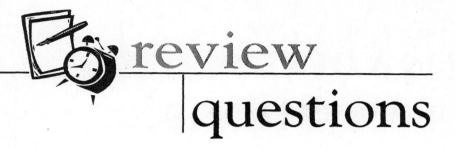

review questions

DIRECTIONS (Questions 1 through 10): Each of the numbered items or incomplete statements in this section is followed by answers or by completions of the statement. Select the ONE lettered answer or completion that is BEST in each case.

1. A green diamond-bordered envelope is considered
   A. first class
   B. second class
   C. third class
   D. fourth class

2. First class mail
   A. must be sealed
   B. must not be sealed
   C. can be inspected
   D. cannot be inspected

3. A Zip code
   A. slows delivery
   B. is always four digits
   C. must be on a line by itself
   D. can be nine digits

4. On an address for automated mailing with the USPS, states should be
   A. written in full
   B. on a separate line
   C. abbreviated in two standard capital letters
   D. abbreviated in two standard lowercase letters

5. For automated processing, the USPS wants all mail to be
   A. punctuated correctly
   B. in italics
   C. in a # 72 font
   D. in all caps

6. The + 4 in a Zip code sorts the mail as to
   A. city
   B. state
   C. county
   D. city block, or large office building

7. When using a data-processing software package, addressing envelopes will usually be found under
   A. "File"
   B. "Edit"
   C. "Tools"
   D. "Save As"

8. The USPS barcode is usually found on the
   A. back of the envelope
   B. return address area
   C. right bottom edge
   D. left bottom edge

9. UPS is another way of sending
   A. e-mail
   B. packages through the USPS
   C. packages through a private service
   D. voice mail

10. Mail must be manually sorted if
    A. in all caps
    B. there is maximum contrast
    C. there is no return address
    D. the address is outside the OCR area

answers & rationales

1.

A. *(Hurlbut, p 1510)*

2.

D. First class can be sealed or not, but it cannot be inspected. *(Fremgen, p 209; USPS)*

3.

D. Zip codes are five digits, and you can add four more totaling nine. It should speed delivery, and it should be on the line with the city and state. *(Lindh, p 277)*

4.

C. For automatic sorting, the United States Postal Service wants states to be standard abbreviations and capitalized. *(Lindh, pp 272, 277; USPS)*

5.

D. For automated sorting at the post office, addresses should not be in italics, or punctuated. A 72 font would be much too large for an envelope. Addresses for automated sorting should be all caps. *(Hurlbut, p 154; USPS)*

6.

D. The +4 sorts the mail into city blocks or large offices. *(USPS)*

7.

C. Under "Tools," you will find envelopes and labels. *(self)*

8.

C. The bar code for automated sorting will be found on the bottom right edge of the envelope. *(Hurlbut, p 154; USPS)*

9.

C. United Parcel Service is a private mailing source for parcels. *(Kinn, p 159)*

10.

D. To be automated, the post office likes mail to be in all caps, with maximum contrast, and inside the optical character reader area. If the address is outside the OCR area, the address cannot be scanned. *(USPS)*

10

Appointment Processes

contents

I. SCHEDULES

A. *Open office booking:* **no appointment necessary; patients can come in at any time the office is open**
   1. Most common appointment system for emergency medical centers
   2. Will be triaged (prioritized) according to severity, acuteness, pain, life-threatening cases

B. *Time-specified appointments:* **each patient is given a certain time to arrive**

C. *Wave scheduling:* **more than one patient is given a time on the hour to come, but then patients are seen on a first come, first served basis. Duration of patients' total appointments is equal to or less than an hour.**
   1. Allowance for early and late arrivals
   2. Attempt to start and finish each hour on time

D. *Double booking:* **two people given the same appointment time**
   1. Not a good practice; duration of the patients' total appointment time is more than the time available on appointment book

E. **Patient's total waiting time should be no more than 20 minutes**
   1. Sign-in sheet made available with times checked by staff frequently
   2. Sign should be posted at the front desk requesting patient to alert staff if the wait is more than 20 minutes or other specified time. Patients do not like to wait!

F. **Blank spaces should be left in the schedule for work-ins, emergencies, and so on**
   1. Work-ins usually handled before lunch and in the late afternoon
   2. If there are no work-ins, the time is used to catch up on the schedule

G. *Categorizing appointments:* **doctors may wish to see all surgery patients on one day or all routine physicals on one afternoon**
   1. Categorizing some appointments (EKGs, sigmoidoscopy) may depend on available facilities and equipment

II. GUIDELINES

A. **Familiarization with types of appointments, treatments and their duration, and doctors' individual habits is necessary to schedule effectively**

B. **Familiarization with facilities, specialty examination rooms, and equipment is needed**

C. Matrix (cross out times for vacations, surgery, meetings, lunch, etc.) must be established before making appointments

D. Missed and canceled appointments should be noted on the patient's chart with the reason

E. Attempts to reschedule missed and canceled appointments should be made with notation on the chart that rescheduling attempts were made

F. *Information necessary to write down for each appointment:* name, phone number, and chief complaint
   1. Ask spelling of name and for what reason they wish to be seen. Repeat phone number (and appointment date and time) for good communication.

G. *Miscellaneous information needed:* whether established or new patient, whether referred and by whom, date of birth, chart number, and address

H. *Doctor delays:* always explain to the patient and give them a choice to reschedule or wait

I. *Emergencies:* must triage and see according to severity

J. *Patient need vs. preference for appointment time:* best to schedule for the patient's convenience unless another time is better (e.g., equipment needed for the patient will be in use; a diabetic patient should be seen soon after eating unless scheduled for specific testing)

K. *Cancellation list:* keep on hand so that schedule can be filled
   1. Try to reschedule every time a patient cancels. Mark cancellations and attempts to reschedule in patient's chart.

L. *Doctor referrals:* to be seen as soon as possible
   1. Referrals out
      a. Make appointments with other facilities while patient is in your office
      b. Log all outside appointments to keep up with outstanding test results

M. *Priority appointments:* keep list on hand

N. *Tickler files:* use for reminders to call patients or check test results that are logged but not yet received

O. *New patient brochure:* send when appointing new patients to inform about the practice and its doctors

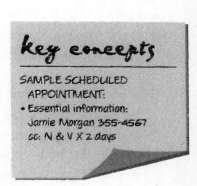

key concepts

SAMPLE SCHEDULED APPOINTMENT:
• Essential information:
Jamie Morgan 355-4567
cc: N & V X 2 days

review questions

DIRECTIONS (Questions 1 through 10): Each of the numbered items or incomplete statements in this section is followed by answers or by completions of the statement. Select the ONE lettered answer or completion that is BEST in each case.

---

1. When setting up the appointment book or the appointment software, you must first "establish the matrix," which is
   A. writing a list of duration for each procedure
   B. deciding how many months ahead you will make appointments
   C. crossing out times that are unavailable for appointments
   D. setting up times for double-booking

2. With open booking, patients are best seen by the doctor
   A. any time—day or night
   B. according to time-specified appointments
   C. in triaged order
   D. in order of time of arrival

3. With wave scheduling, patients are given appointment times
   A. every 15–20 minutes
   B. at the same hour, even though the total allotted time is not enough to see both patients
   C. according to the type of appointment they have (for example, all B/P checks)
   D. at the same hour, but the total time needed for both appointments will be allotted.

4. Good managers will assume that
   A. patients do not mind waiting as long as the doctor spends enough time with each patient when they are seen
   B. there should be no blank spaces in the appointment book
   C. patients do not mind delays if there is an emergency
   D. there will be times needed in appointment schedules for emergencies

5. To have an efficient daily schedule, the medical assistant making the appointments should
   A. leave blank spaces for work-ins when patients cancel
   B. set up several specialty procedures such as EKGs or sigmoidoscopies within an hour
   C. be familiar with duration of clinical procedures and treatments
   D. ignore doctor's habits and pace of seeing patients

6. When scheduling appointments, which of the following information can wait until the patient arrives?
   A. allergies
   B. name of patient
   C. phone number
   D. chief complaint

7. When a patient cancels an appointment, it is good practice to
   A. ask them to call back later to reschedule
   B. note it in their chart and reschedule the appointment then
   C. write on your tickler file to call the patient and reschedule
   D. refer them to another doctor

8. A patient has called to make an appointment. Of the following first responses, which is appropriate?
   A. "When would you like to be seen?"
   B. "For what reason do you need to be seen?"
   C. "What's your problem?"
   D. "Do you have any insurance?"

9. Of the following chief complaints, which would you triage last?
   A. nausea and vomiting
   B. chronic cough
   C. acute stomach cramps
   D. sprained wrist

10. Appointments for referrals to other doctors are best made
    A. by the patient
    B. by the doctor
    C. while the patient is in your office
    D. by calling the patient after the patient has time to return home

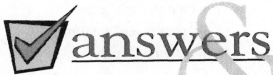

answers & rationales

1.

C. Although writing a list of procedures and the time each one takes is a must in making appointments, a is not the correct answer. Establishing the matrix is the first thing you do when you begin a new start for appointments. It means that the first thing is to cross out all times the doctor will be unavailable for appointments. Cross out vacation days, holidays, times the doctor is gone for surgery or rounds, etc. Once you know the unavailable times, you can begin to make appointments in the available spaces. As for d, you will never set up times to double-book. You try to set aside times for work-ins and emergencies so that you will not have to double-book. *(Fremgen, p 155)*

2.

C. When you have open booking, patients do not have to have appointments to be seen. They walk in and are seen according to the most urgent appointments first; otherwise they will be seen in order of arrival. In other words, a patient arriving with severe bleeding will be escorted to the exam room before a patient with a bad cold. *(Kinn, p 121)*

3.

D. In wave scheduling, each hour is supposed to start and end on time. You will allot a certain number of patients each hour but their appointments added together will not take up more than the total hour. All of these patients will be told to come in at the beginning of the hour, but will then be seen in order of arrival. This will help account for patients who are early and late. *(Hurlbut, p 159)*

4.

D. Always set aside time for work-ins and emergencies. Blank spaces should be left just before lunch and at the end of each day. This will be catch up time. Each practice should evaluate schedules periodically to see if they are leaving too much or too little time. As far as answers a and c, patients are consumers of a service. More and more the public is demanding fair treatment concerning their time. This means the consumer's time is just as sacred as the doctor's time. *(Kinn, p 126)*

5.

C. To effectively make appointments, the medical assistant has to know how long procedures take, how many specialty rooms are available, how long it takes to clean equipment, and such. Unless there are a lot of equipment and specialty machines on hand, it will take too long to clean a scope to schedule several in one hour. Spaces for work-ins will be left daily, not just when patients cancel appointments. When patients cancel, there should be a waiting list of patients who would like to be seen sooner than their appointed times. *(Kinn, pp 124–6)*

6.

A. Allergies do not have to be given on the phone when scheduling an appointment. That can wait until the patient is giving a medical history. When scheduling an appointment, however, you must have the patient's name, phone number, and chief complaint (so you will know how much time to allow for the appointment). *(Hurlbut, p 158)*

7.

B. When a patient cancels, you should make an attempt right then to reschedule. Note the cancellation, reason, and rescheduled appointment on their chart. If for some reason the patient cannot reschedule when they cancel, find out why, note it all on the patient's chart, and for good measure, have them call you back, but also note on your calendar to call them and reschedule. You can never have too many checks and balances in the medical office. *(Fremgen, pp 156–57)*

8.

B. "For what reason do you need to be seen" is specific and professional. As for answer a, you want to be more specific when appointing patients. Ask them if they prefer mornings or afternoons, and give them two available times to choose from once they tell you their morning or afternoon preference. You could go back and forth all day saying "when would you like to be seen" if you are not specific. "What's your problem?" sounds too abrupt and snippy. "Do you have any insurance?" as the first question you ask, sounds as if you are only interested in patients who can afford to be seen. *(Kinn, pp 128–29)*

9.

B. Most problems that are acute, painful, or an emergency should be seen first. Nausea and vomiting could lead to dehydration; in c the stomach cramps are acute, and a sprained wrist is usually painful. The fact that the cough is chronic lets you know it can wait—unless it has become much worse lately and includes shortness of breath. This is where the right questions have to be asked by the triage personnel. *(Fremgen, p 152)*

10.

C. It is most efficient to make the appointment when the patient is right there in your office. By having the patient there, you can consult with them about available times and get directions or questions answered. Usually, the doctor will not make the appointment, but may wish to speak to the other doctor after the appointment is made. It may be hard for the patient to make the appointment because of questions about diagnosis and reasons for referral. Many times, after the patient leaves it is hard to reach them. Your least busy times may be when the patient is away from home, and it often is much more time-consuming when you have to call two and three times to connect with the patient. *(Kinn, p 134–35)*

11

Community Services

I. RESOURCES

Find available community resources by checking local libraries, telephone books, and agencies like the public health department and social services.

A. Hospitals
1. **General hospitals:** short-term hospitalization
2. **Specialty hospitals:** hospitalization for specific diseases such as cancer and tuberculosis, or for psychiatric care

B. *Surgical centers:* usually for outpatient surgeries

C. *Emergency medical centers:* smaller than hospital emergency areas, usually for minor trauma

D. *Convalescent care:* nursing homes, usually for long-term geriatric (elderly) care

E. *Clinics:* various specialties in one office complex

F. *Home health care agencies:* for patient care in the home

G. *Senior day care:* elderly sitting services

H. *Health department:* preventive health care, promotion of disease control, and public health education

I. *Social services department:* financial aid and human resource aid (e.g., Medicaid, food stamps, adult protection, child protection, abuse, adoption)

J. *Volunteer agencies and support groups:* medical assistants should be familiar with their own community resources for referrals when needed for financial, emotional, or other kinds of support
1. **American Cancer Society:** education, health fair participation, and cancer prevention
2. **American Red Cross:** blood drives, emergency services, CPR classes
3. **American Heart Association:** wellness education, prevention of heart disease like MI (myocardial infarction) or CAD (coronary artery disease), CPR classes
4. **American Diabetes Association:** diabetes education (insulin injections, diabetic retinopathy)
5. **Hospice:** for dying patients and their families
6. **Council on Aging:** home-delivered meals, legal and insurance information, help for neglected seniors, and transportation assistance
7. **Lions Club:** financial support for the visually impaired
8. **Children's services:** help for cases of abuse or neglect and financial assistance

key concepts

- Medical assistants should be knowledgeable about community support groups, clinics and hospitals, emergency services, volunteer organizations, and home health care agencies.

9. **Handicapped and developmental services:** evaluation, management, and rehabilitation

10. **Drug and alcohol abuse services:** education and rehabilitation

11. **Rehabilitation services:** mental, physical, and drug abuse, and cases with vocational and counseling services

12. **American Lung Association:** education, smoking cessation clinics, and support groups for lung cancer, emphysema

13. **Weight control and dietary services:** nutrition education and support groups

14. **Organ procurement agencies:** organize efforts to match organ donors and recipients

15. **AIDS support groups:** for all patients and families

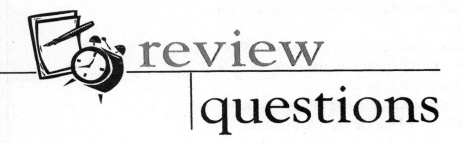

review
questions

DIRECTIONS (Questions 1 through 10): Each of the numbered items or incomplete statements in this section is followed by answers or by completions of the statement. Select the ONE lettered answer or completion that is BEST in each case.

---

1. A person who has macular degeneration would least likely use which of the following services?
   A. Lion's Club
   B. local library
   C. support group for the blind
   D. hospice

2. A person with retinopathy would most likely get help from
   A. hospice
   B. drug and alcohol abuse services
   C. American Cancer Society
   D. American Diabetes Association

3. A person with a terminal illness may get support/help from
   A. bariatrics services
   B. Council on Aging
   C. hospice
   D. rehabilitation services

4. Home-delivered meals might be sought from
   A. American Cancer Society
   B. Council on Aging
   C. weight control and dietary services
   D. American Lung Association

5. Educational pamphlets about emphysema most likely will be published by
   A. rehabilitation services
   B. American Red Cross
   C. American Lung Association

   D. American Heart Association

6. Programs for smoking cessation would most likely be offered by
   A. American Diabetes Association
   B. American Lung Association
   C. rehabilitation services
   D. hospice

7. CPR classes are usually offered by
   A. American Heart Association
   B. children's services
   C. Council on Aging
   D. American Diabetes Association

8. Child abuse cases should be reported to
   A. home health care agencies
   B. Social Services Department
   C. handicapped and developmental services
   D. drug and alcohol abuse services

9. Report communicable diseases to
   A. hospice
   B. health department
   C. children's services
   D. emergency medical centers

10. Adoption information can be sought through
    A. health department
    B. Social Services Department
    C. Lion's Club
    D. children's services

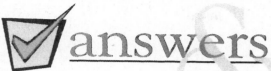

answers & rationales

1.

D. A person with macular degeneration may eventually lose their reading vision. The Lion's Club may sponsor them for special magnifiers; the local library would be a good source for large-print materials and books that are taped; a support group for the blind may eventually be a good resource for emotional needs. Hospice would not be needed, as macular degeneration is not a terminal illness. *(Hurlbut, pp 171–75; self)*

2.

D. A person with retinopathy has the disease usually because of diabetic complications. Therefore, the American Diabetes Association would be the most helpful support service of those listed. *(Hurlbut, pp 171–75; self)*

3.

C. Terminal illnesses are the reason for home health and hospice services. Hospice can provide help for families and patients. Bariatrics is services for the obese; the Council on Aging helps the elderly with meals and other activities of daily living; rehabilitation helps someone regain skills they lost with a disease or accident. *(Hurlbut, pp 171–75; self)*

4.

B. The Council on Aging delivers meals to the elderly who may not be able to cook for themselves. *(Hurlbut, pp 171–75; self)*

5.

C. The American Lung Association would most likely distribute pamphlets about the lung disease, emphysema. *(Hurlbut, pp 171–75; self)*

6.

B. Smoking is one of the main reasons for lung cancers and other lung diseases; therefore, the American Lung Association will often offer smoking cessation support groups. *(Hurlbut, pp 171–75; self)*

7.

A. CPR classes are typically offered by the American Red Cross and the American Heart Association. *(Hurlbut, pp 171–75; self)*

8.

B. All child or elder abuse cases or even suspected cases should be reported to the Social Services Department. *(Hurlbut, pp 171–75; self)*

9.

B. All reportable diseases for each state should be reported to the Health Department, which will report them to the Center for Disease Control. In this way epidemics can hopefully be prevented or at least curbed. *(Hurlbut, pp 171–5; self)*

10.

B. There are private adoption agencies, but publicly, the Department of Social Services handles adoptions. *(Hurlbut, pp 171–75; self)*

CHAPTER

12

Office Management

contents

I. EDITORIAL AND TRAVEL DUTIES

A. Office library

1. Physician's journals
   a. **JAMA (Journal of the American Medical Association)**
   b. Specialty journals
2. Patient educational materials
   a. Videos
   b. Disease brochures
   c. Models
3. Organization
   a. **Card catalog:** author, title, and subject
   b. Abstracts may summarize and file the most important points of an article
   c. Journals bound and index of contents made

B. Research

1. Materials search
   a. Card catalog
   b. Periodical index **(Index Medicus)**
   c. Computer search
   d. Bibliography list

C. Speech typing

1. Double-spaced

D. *Arrangement of meetings:* **block out meetings on the appointment schedule and reschedule appointments if necessary, or assign coverage for those attending the meetings.**

1. Reason for meeting
2. Place
3. Time
4. Date
5. Duration
6. Expected attendance
7. Announcement of meeting
8. Food requirements (refreshments or meals)
9. **Agenda:** items to be discussed at the meeting
10. Minute taking
    a. Presider
    b. Name of association
    c. Date, time, place, and type of meeting
    d. Those present
    e. Minutes read and approved
    f. Items of business, and any motions made and by whom made

    g. Hour of adjournment

    h. Programs or speeches are not summarized

E. *Travel arrangements:* block out times for travel on the appointment schedule and assign coverage or reschedule appointments.

    1. Preparation of itinerary

    2. Motel reservations, confirmation of reservations, and late arrival guarantee (credit card needed)

    3. Method of transportation

    4. Date and time of departure and return

    5. Purchase of necessary tickets

    6. Mailing of necessary registration

    7. Inclusion of maps, brochures, other necessary information

F. Patient instruction and information booklets

    1. Booklets updated and sent to patients to introduce them to the practice or to acquaint them with their diseases

II. POLICIES AND PROCEDURES/OFFICE MANAGEMENT

A. Policy manual/personnel

    1. Philosophy of office

    2. Line-of-authority chart—who reports to whom

    3. Policies of the office

        a. **Interviewing, hiring, and firing**

- Knowledge of fair employment practice laws is necessary
- Same questions should be asked of each interviewee so that a fair evaluation can be made
- All applicants should be notified when positions are filled or given an approximate date when filled
- Exit interviews should be conducted when employees leave
- Warnings and documentation should be provided during evaluations so that the employees may have a chance to improve unless circumstances (e.g., stealing, insubordination) require immediate dismissal

        b. **Sick leave and vacation:** established policies are necessary for all employees

        c. **Evaluation of personnel**

- Probationary period: a specific period of time before the employee is hired permanently
- Documentation of all evaluations
- Regular reviews
- Evaluations to be reviewed and signed by reviewer and reviewee

        d. **Dress code:** should be established and adhered to

e. **Other office management**
- Staff meetings when necessary
- Harmony of staff included in management
- Work flow/patient flow: manager monitors equality of work-load and flow of patients and makes changes when necessary

4. **Office maintenance:** equipment justification, ordering, and maintenance, and housekeeping

B. Procedure manual

1. **Job descriptions:** can consult DOT (Dictionary of Occupational Titles)
2. Step-by-step guide for carrying out each job in the office
3. Guide for the clinical setups (minor surgery setups, specialty procedures, and so on)

III. ACCOUNTING/FINANCIAL MANAGEMENT

A. Payroll

1. Employee information
   a. Name
   b. Social Security number
   c. Exemptions and deductions
   d. Gross salary (before taxes) or hourly wage
   e. Amount of overtime if applicable
   f. Marital status and length of pay period (for income tax withheld)
2. Forms
   a. **W-4 form:** withholding allowance certificate; shows the number of exemptions claimed
   b. **W-2 form:** wage and tax statement; given at the end of the year or by January 31 at the latest
   c. **Form 941:** employer's quarterly federal tax return
   d. **Form 940:** employer's annual federal unemployment tax return (FUTA)
3. Taxes
   a. **FICA:** Federal Insurance Contributions Act
      - **OASI:** Old Age and Survivors Insurance
      - **HI:** hospitalization under Medicare
      - **DI:** disability insurance
   b. **FUTA:** Federal Unemployment Tax Act
   c. **FWT:** Federal withholding tax
   d. **SWT:** State withholding tax
   e. Local taxes in some areas

B. Bank reconciliation

1. Monthly bank statement

---

key concepts

- Every office must have a policy manual and a procedure manual.

key concepts

- The AAMA certified medical assistant must recertify every five years by obtaining sixty CEUs or by retesting.

key concepts

- You cannot use the certification title (CMA) of the AAMA when expired without re-certification.

2. Reconciliation of bank statement with checkbook balance
3. Subtract bank fees (service charges, etc.) from checkbook balance and circle this figure as reconciliation 1
4. Subtract outstanding checks from bank statement balance and add outstanding deposits to bank statement balance. Circle this figure as reconciliation 2
5. Reconciliations 1 and 2 should be the same

C. Check writing

1. Stub of each check should have amount, date, payee, and purpose of the check
2. Stub is filled out before removing the check
3. Check is voided if a mistake has been made
4. Acceptance of checks
   a. All spaces filled out correctly
   b. Third-party checks accepted only for payments by insurance companies
   c. Checks accepted only for the amount due and correct date
   d. Acceptance of no check marked "payment in full" unless it is, in fact, full payment
   e. **Endorsement:** on the back of the check write "for deposit only" to ensure that the check can only be deposited into the proper account

D. Deposits to account

1. Currency (paper money) listed first; face side up with larger bills on top and like denominations together
2. Coin amount listed
3. Checks recorded individually by ABA number (the fraction in the right upper corner) and amount of check
4. Money orders and other types of payments recorded last

E. Accounts payable

1. Bills paid by the physician's office are usually paid by check
2. **Invoice (not a bill):** shows amount due and describes item
3. **Statement:** bill for goods and materials received
4. **Petty cash:** small amount of cash to have on hand for expenses and bills too small to require checks; instead one check is written "To Petty Cash" and the money put in a cash drawer to pay small bills

F. Accounts receivable

1. **Amounts patients owe the physician:** best kept to minimum by collecting on day of service
2. **Extending credit:** if amount to be paid is in more than four installments, a truth-in-lending statement must be signed (states whether or not interest will be charged)

key concepts

SAMPLE POLICIES FOUND IN POLICY MANUAL:
1. All employees will have a paid Christmas vacation.
2. All employees will be evaluated three times a year.

key concepts

• Accounts receivable are balances that have not yet been paid by patients.
• Accounts payable are balances that are owed by the medical office to others.

3. **Credit cards:** frequently accepted in the doctor's office for payments on a bill

4. **Insurance payments:** patient must sign a record release form (patient is giving consent for the insurance company to know confidential information so that payment can be authorized) and Assignment of Benefits Form (so that payment will be made directly to the physician)

5. **Cycle billing:** sending bills at different times of the month for smooth cash flow
   Example: send A to E on the first of the month; send F to J on the sixth; and send K to O on the twelfth

6. **Delinquent accounts:** 120 days overdue or according to office policy; may be turned over to a collection agency
   a. Collection letters may be sent, and telephone calls made without harassment
   b. Requests for payment usually at 30, 60, and 90 days overdue
   c. Accounts sent to collection agency are flagged so that no more bills will be sent to the patient by the office

7. **Collection ratio:** total payments YTD (year to date) divided by charges YTD, less adjustments; should be approximately 95 percent

8. **Accounts receivable ratio:** accounts receivable balance divided by average gross monthly charges equals the average number of months in which accounts are being paid; should be less than two months
   a. Aging of accounts should be done monthly to increase collections efforts

9. **Pegboard system:** "write it once"
   a. Superbill (charge slip, encounter form, receipt), ledger card, and journal (daysheet entry) all done at one time
   b. "Write it once" due to use of pegboard, shingled forms, ledger cards, and carbon transfers
   c. Computerized office equipment now replacing pegboard systems

IV. INVENTORY

A. *Yearly:* for tax and depreciation purposes

B. *Daily:* for ordering supplies as needed

C. *Budget:* duty of management to evaluate needed equipment, justify need, and budget accordingly

V. PHYSICAL PLANT

A. Maintenance of equipment, repairs of physical plant, safety of office, and so on, are all part of management

VI. LIABILITY COVERAGE

A. Coverage for doctors and employees is a necessity

B. Policies kept indefinitely

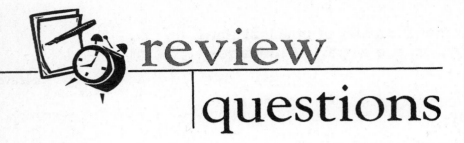
DIRECTIONS (Questions 1 through 10): Each of the numbered items or incomplete statements in this section is followed by answers or by completions of the statement. Select the ONE lettered answer or completion that is BEST in each case.

1. One of the most important physician journals arriving at the medical office is
   A. PMA
   B. Index Medicus
   C. JAMA
   D. PDR

2. An important writing/organizational skill the medical assistant needs to summarize important articles is
   A. binding magazines
   B. composing abstracts
   C. organizing a card catalog
   D. writing agendas

3. To report on a past medical meeting, the medical assistant will need to know how to
   A. prepare an itinerary
   B. write an agenda
   C. write minutes
   D. write a bibliography

4. When arranging meetings, the least important information needed is the
   A. place of meeting
   B. time and date of meeting
   C. guest list
   D. weather report

5. When taking minutes, it is not required to report the
   A. date, time, and place of meeting
   B. name of the presider
   C. motions made and by whom
   D. summarized points of the program if one is given

6. To guarantee a motel room for your doctor when he attends a medical convention, you must have
   A. an itinerary
   B. a hard copy of the reservation
   C. given the motel the doctor's credit card number
   D. given the time of arrival

7. A line-of-authority chart is needed to
   A. find out who you will need to bypass to get the job done
   B. let all employees know who has the most power in the office
   C. let each employee know who gets paid the most
   D. designate who is responsible for whom and to whom each person reports

8. The DOT would most likely be used when organizing a
   A. policy manual
   B. procedure manual

C. patient brochure

D. bank reconciliation

9. When interviewing a potential employee for the first time,

A. you can ask them anything you think is necessary to evaluate them

B. you will probably tell them the salary they will be receiving if hired

C. you should ask the same questions as you do of all other applicants

D. you should find out if they are pregnant or considering becoming pregnant before hiring them

10. Each employee should be granted sick leave according to

A. their age and sex

B. seniority

C. pre-established policies

D. favoritism

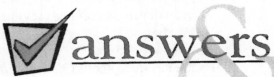

answers & rationales

1.

C. The only physician journal listed is the JAMA, the Journal of the American Medical Association. The PMA is the Professional Medical Assistant's journal and the PDR is the Physician's Desk Reference, a reference book of medications. The Index Medicus is found in the library to use for looking up articles. *(Kinn, p 340)*

2.

B. Writing abstracts is the same thing as summarizing magazine articles. Doctors may mark in their magazines those articles for the medical assistant to summarize and file for future reference. *(Hurlbut, p 172)*

3.

C. When attending meetings, someone is designated to take minutes that summarize the business that goes on in the meeting. Itineraries are prepared for people taking a trip, and agendas are written to state the topics that will be covered at a meeting. A bibliography is a list of books used as a reference. *(Kinn, p 350)*

4.

D. Though the weather report is important in planning a meeting, meetings should be planned enough in advance that the weather report a few weeks or months ahead may not be the same as predicted; therefore, the date, time, and place of the meeting and the guest list will be more important. *(Kinn, p 350)*

5.

D. Correct minutes report the time, date, and place of the meeting, the name of the presider, the motions that are made and who made them. The points of a program or speech do not have to be summarized. *(Kinn, p 350)*

6.

C. You are guaranteeing a room because you do not know for sure what time the doctor will arrive. Some motels will cancel your reservation after 6 P.M. if you have not guaranteed the room. To guarantee it, you must give a credit card number. *(self)*

7.

D. A line of authority chart does not state who has the most power or who gets paid the most. Professionals will not bypass someone on the line of authority until they have gone through the line appropriately and exhausted all resources. The line of authority chart does designate whom each person reports to and whom each person is responsible for. *(Kinn, p 364)*

8.

B. The Dictionary of Occupational Titles is used to designate duties for jobs and job descriptions. Therefore, when writing procedures for each job, the DOT would be very helpful. *(Kinn, p 366)*

9.

C. To be nondiscriminatory, each interviewee should be asked the very same questions. This will give a fair comparison of all applicants. Certain personal questions cannot be asked such as pregnancy, religion, etc. Usually salaries are not disclosed until closer to the actual choosing of an applicant. *(Kinn, p 271)*

10.

C. All facilities should have a policy manual that discloses dress codes, sick leave, benefits, etc. These policies may take into account seniority, but would be discriminating if age, sex, or favoritism would be a criterion for sick leave. *(Kinn, p 365)*

13 Health Insurance

contents

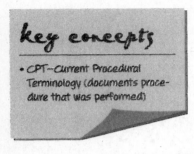

key concepts

• CPT—Current Procedural Terminology (documents procedure that was performed)

I. INSURANCE TERMINOLOGY

A. *Assignment of benefits:* specification of whom is to receive payment; if the patient signs a form assigning benefits to the doctor, the payment from the insurance company will be sent to the doctor

B. *Deductible:* predetermined amount to be paid "out of pocket" by the patient before insurance will begin to pay. If the deductible is $75.00, the patient must pay the first $75.00 of the bill; then the insurance will begin to pay its percentage

C. *Co-payment:* a designated amount or rate the patient must pay toward the bill; after the deductible has been met, the patient may have a $10.00 co-payment on each service thereafter or may pay a certain percentage of the bill

D. *Fee schedule:* a list of the fees charged for each service

E. *Usual fee:* the most prevalent fee doctors charge for each procedure

F. *Customary fees:* a range of fees that many doctors in a locale charge for each procedure

G. *Reasonable fees:* fees charged a patient when circumstances make the usual procedure more complicated

H. *Precertification:* prior authorization by an insurance company for payment for a specified procedure in the hospital

I. *DRG (diagnostic related groups):* three-digit numbering system for payment purposes, puts related diagnoses into groups according to procedures performed, patient's age, sex, discharge status, and complications/comorbidities

J. *Coordination of benefits:* if a patient is insured by more than one insurance company, the primary insurance company will pay first, the secondary insurance company will pay on the amount left, and so on; however, the total of all payments should be no more than 100 percent of the charges

II. TYPES OF INSURANCE

A. *Medicaid:* provides health care for the indigent
   1. Cards may be issued monthly so cards should be checked for current date (varies from state to state)

B. *Medicare:* two parts
   1. **Hospital (Part A):** those receiving Social Security benefits automatically receive hospital benefits under Medicare
   2. **Medical (Part B):** If a person receives Part A, she/he is eligible (there are others that may be eligible as well), but all must pay the premium monthly

C. *CHAMPUS:* Civilian Health and Medical Program of the Uniformed Services

D. *CHAMPVA:* Civilian Health and Medical Program of the Veterans Administration

E. *Blue Cross and Blue Shield:* medical and surgical insurance
   1. **Blue Cross:** hospitalization
   2. **Blue Shield:** physician's payments

F. *Workers' compensation:* covers the patient for loss of wages and provides health care when illness or injury is job related
   1. Doctor must file "Doctor's First Report of Occupational Injury" within 72 hours of the patient's first visit

key concepts

• ICD-9—International Classification of Diseases, Ninth Edition (documents the patient's diagnosis or disease)

III. FILING OF CLAIMS

A. Universal Claim Form: HCFA-1500
   1. First form completed without charge
   2. **Multiple forms:** justifiable for physician's office to charge for completion
   3. **Authorization to release information:** must be signed to give the office permission to release patient's confidential information
   4. **Assignment of benefits:** must be signed for payment to be sent directly to the provider
      a. "Signature on file": tailor-made document to file in patient's permanent chart stating release of records to insurance company and benefits assigned to provider
   5. Diagnostic codes must be correct and agree with procedure codes, and vice versa
   6. Dates should have six-digit format, 00/00/00
   7. Upgrading of knowledge of insurance codes and formats is a must for good reimbursement

B. Electronic claims filing

C. Rejections
   1. Diagnosis and treatment may not be relevant
   2. Incomplete forms

3. Inaccurate coding
4. Items incorrectly typed, such as date 10-1-00 not typed as 10-01-00

D. Coding

1. ICD-9-CM: *International Classification of Diseases,* Ninth Edition, *Clinical Modification,* three volumes
   a. **Diseases:** tabular list
   b. **Diseases:** alphabetic index
   c. **Procedures:** tabular list and alphabetic index (not used in the physician's office)
   d. **Three-digit code that codes individual diseases:** add decimal and extra digits to code specificities about each disease.
2. CPT-4: *Current Procedural Terminology,* five sections
   a. Medicine (evaluation and management codes located here— new patient codes start with 99201)
   b. Anesthesiology—starts with "0"
   c. Surgery—starts with "3"
   d. Radiology—starts with "7"
   e. Pathology and laboratory
   f. **Five-digit code that codes medical procedures:** add decimal and two digit modifier to show that a procedure has been altered
      • -50—modifier meaning bilateral procedure
      • -51—modifier meaning multiple procedures
      • -99—modifier meaning multiple modifiers
3. HCPCS: Health Care Financing Administration Common Procedure Coding System
   a. Five-digit Medicare alphanumeric codes based on CPT codes
   b. Three levels of coding
4. Superbills/encounter forms
   a. A listing of codes of possible services rendered
      • Diagnosis is entered, services rendered are circled, patient data is entered, and fees are entered
      • May be tailor-made for each practice to list most often performed procedures and codes
   b. **Completed superbill:** can sometimes be attached to the insurance form for filing the claim

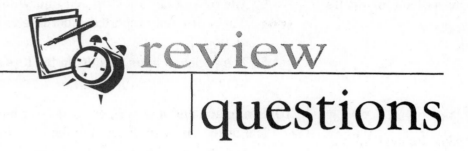

review questions

DIRECTIONS (Questions 1 through 10): Each of the numbered items or incomplete statements in this section is followed by answers or by completions of the statement. Select the ONE lettered answer or completion that is BEST in each case.

---

1. Signing a HCFA-1500 form that designates the doctor to receive payment from the insurance company is
   A. assignment of benefits
   B. release of records
   C. coordination of benefits
   D. precertification

2. Coding-related diagnoses and procedures is necessary to
   A. file insurance
   B. receive an insurance payment for a service
   C. receive a personal payment from a patient
   D. have a deductible paid by a patient

3. A service covered without a deductible requires
   A. that a patient pay a certain amount before insurance will pay
   B. no payment from the patient for the service to be paid
   C. no premium to be paid
   D. 20% to be paid by the patient

4. Precertification for a procedure means the patient must
   A. get a second opinion
   B. have a secondary insurance
   C. have prior authorization from the insurance company before the procedure is performed
   D. first certify the insurance premiums have been paid

5. DRGs (Diagnostic-Related Groups) organizes payment for related diagnoses according to
   A. whether or not a patient can pay personally
   B. surgical complications, age, and secondary diagnoses
   C. alphabetical order
   d. necessary labwork

6. A patient who has met her deductible still has to pay $10.00 when she checks out. This payment is called the
   A. usual fee
   B. co-payment
   C. customary fee
   D. interest

7. In order for two insurance companies to pay no more than 100% of a bill, there may be a/an
   A. coordination of benefits clause
   B. precertification
   C. fee schedule
   D. assignment of benefits

8. Anyone who has Medicare will automatically receive
   A. Part A Hospitalization
   B. Part B Medical
   C. Part C Laboratory
   D. Part D Funeral expense

9. Worker's compensation pays the medical bill only when
   A. The patient is injured at work and has been working at least 2 years
   B. A patient working for a big company gets injured at home or at work

C. The patient has a job-related injury/illness that is officially reported according to regulations
D. The patient's injury results in the loss of a limb

10. Evaluation and management codes for medical office visits are located in the
    A. ICD-9 book, "Pathology" section
    B. "Medicine" section of the CPT-4 book
    C. "Surgery" section of the CPT-4 book
    D. "Medicine" section of the ICD-9 book

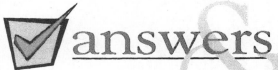

answers & rationales

1.

A. An assignment of benefits is signed so that the doctor receives the check for services rendered instead of the patient's receiving the check. *(Fremgen, pp 316–19)*

2.

B. If a procedure and a diagnosis are not related so that the procedure is done because of the diagnosis, the insurance will not pay. *(Lindh, pp 329–32)*

3.

B. If a service requires no deductible and is paid 100%, the patient will not have to pay anything. *(Fremgen, p 309)*

4.

C. Some procedures may not be covered generally by an insurance company, but, because of certain circumstances, may actually be covered with prior authorization. This is called precertification. *(Lindh, p 319)*

5.

B. Certain procedures may be covered for a certain number of days usually, but, because of the patient's age or other complications, may require more days to recover. DRGs organize diagnoses according to these factors. *(Kinn, p 336)*

6.

B. Many insurances require certain co-payments. The deductible still must be met, but each time a service is rendered a certain amount of money may be required. For instance, some insurance covers medications. After deductibles have been met, patients may only have to pay $10.00 for every medicine they buy even though the medicine may cost more. Sometimes the co-payment may be different depending on whether or not the drug is generic. *(Lindh, p 318)*

7.

A. Coordination of benefits means that if a person has more than one insurance, one will be primary (paying the most, usually 80% of the assigned amount) and one may be secondary (20% of the assigned amount), but neither will pay an amount that will make the total paid more than 100%. *(Lindh, p 318)*

8.

A. Part A, Hospitalization, is automatically received by those with Medicare. Patients can elect to pay for Part B if they want it. There is no Part C or D. *(Lindh, p 307)*

9.

C. To receive worker's compensation, you must officially report the injury within 24 hours, and it must be a job-related injury or disease. *(Hurlbut, p 203)*

10.

B. E and M codes are located in the beginning of the CPT code book. These codes are for new and established office visits. Other codes for labwork or surgery may be found in other sections of the book. *(Hurlbut, p 299)*

SECTION III

Clinical Procedures

14 Infection Control

contents

I. MEDICAL ASEPSIS

A. *Clean technique (as free of bacteria as possible): used during noninvasive procedures*

1. **Handwashing:** the single most important method of medical asepsis
   a. Wash hands thoroughly (may leave on plain gold band) with fingertips downward
2. **Sanitization:** washing of items with detergent and water or antiseptic (used on living tissue)
3. **Disinfection:** destroying many infectious organisms using chemicals (used on inanimate objects)
4. Chain of transmission
   a. **Reservoir host:** provides nourishment for infection
   b. **Means of exit:** infectious organism exits through open wound or other body orifice
   c. **Transmission:** to another susceptible host through contact with a person or a person's infected waste or discharge (sneeze, feces) or contaminated objects
   d. **Means of entry:** infectious organism gains entry through the skin or a body orifice
5. Breaking the chain
   a. Removal of nourishment necessary for infectious organisms to live
      • Decrease oxygen if organism thrives on it
      • Change temperature if organism thrives at certain temperatures
      • Decrease moisture if organism thrives in a wet or moist environment
      • Increase light if organism thrives in darkness
   b. Immunizations
6. Universal blood and body fluid precautions
   a. **Barrier protection:** masks, gloves, gowns, aprons, and goggles
   b. Never recap contaminated needles

B. **Guarding against infectious agents**

1. Bacteria: classified by morphology (size and shape)
   a. **Cocci:** round-shaped
   b. **Staphylococci:** round clusters of bacteria
   c. **Streptococci:** round bacteria in chains
   d. **Diplococci:** round bacteria in twos
   e. **Spirilla:** spiral-shaped bacterial
   f. **Bacilli:** rod-shaped bacteria
   g. **Chlamydia:** small bacteria that cannot live without a host
2. **Fungi:** yeasts and molds; vegetative organisms
3. **Rickettsiae:** parasites causing spotted fever and typhus
4. **Protozoa:** single-celled animals, usually nonparasitic

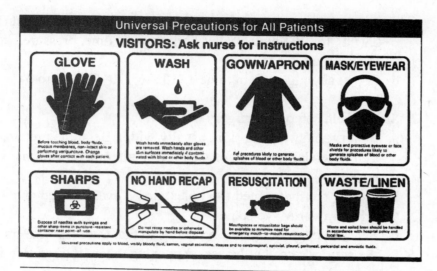

FIGURE 14–1 Universal precautions for all patients for the protection of patients, family, and health care workers.

5. **Helminths:** parasitic worms
6. **Virus:** smaller than the microorganisms listed above

C. Medical examination instruments

1. **Otoscope:** for viewing the ear
2. **Ophthalmoscope:** for viewing the eye
3. **Stethoscope:** auscultation (listening) of heart, lungs, bowel sounds, and bruits (abnormal sounds); listening to the brachial artery during blood pressure checks
4. **Tuning fork:** checks sound perception (air and bone conduction)
5. **Reflex/percussion hammer:** checks reflexes (knee jerk, ankle jerk, brachioradialis, biceps, and triceps)
6. **Pinwheel:** checks sensations
7. **Laryngeal mirror:** views back of throat, tonsils, and adenoids
8. **Speculum:** opens area for viewing, inspection, examination, and passing instruments
    a. Vaginal
    b. Nasal
    c. Proctoscope
    d. Anoscope
9. **Lister bandage scissors:** cut through bandages; have blunt, rounded end

II. SURGICAL ASEPSIS

A. Guarding against infectious microorganisms during surgical or invasive techniques

1. **Sterilization:** complete destruction of all microorganisms, including spores

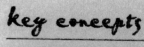

key concepts

• The larger the number suture, the smaller the suture is. Example: 10-0 is thinner than 5-0.

a. **Autoclave** (e.g., pressurized steam at 15 pounds of pressure, 250° F, for 20 minutes): has variations of time, pressure, and temperature
b. **Dry heat:** subject to high heat (165 to 170° C for 2 to 3 hours)

2. Sterile field setup and surgery
   a. **Skin prep:** swabbing skin, usually with a Betadine preparation to render it as free of pathogenic microorganisms as possible
   b. Sterile, nonfenestrated (no holes) drape over cleaned and dried tray or Mayo stand
   c. Fenestrated drape (has a hole in it so that the drape covers the surgical area but leaves an opening where the incision is to be made)
   d. All supplies, such as gauze sponges, sutures, needle holders, forceps, scissors, scalpels, cotton-tipped applicators, and cautery, must be sterile and "popped onto" or transferred to sterile field
      • Reaching over the sterile field = contamination
      • Anything below waist level is considered nonsterile
      • Anything touching outside a 1-inch border = contamination
      • Wetting of sterile field = contamination (unless it has a plastic barrier)
   e. Gloves, gown, masks, and any other barriers needed are set aside for donning by the doctor and assistants
      • Surgical scrub is necessary for the doctor and any assistants
      • Hands and arms are washed and scrubbed up to the elbows for a prescribed amount of time, fingernails are cleaned, and fingertips are held upward
      • No jewelry is worn
   f. Light is in place and waste receptacles (puncture-proof containers) available for needles and other sharps; hazardous materials bags available for contaminated disposables
   g. Receptacle used for soaking contaminated instruments so that blood will not dry
   h. Sterile transfer forceps used if it is necessary to move sterile items
      • Sides of container not covered with disinfecting solution must not be touched when removing forceps
      • Sterile gauze is used to wipe instrument dry after rinsing with sterile water

B. *Surgical instruments:* **must be sterile if used invasively in the body**

---

key concepts

• Clinical equipment that comes in contact with a patient should be cleaned between patients, unless the contact was invasive; then the parts of the equipment that contacted the patient should be sterilized.

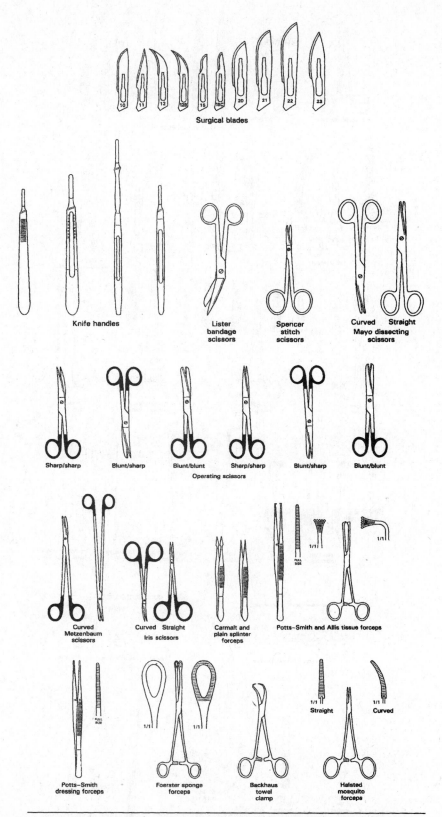

FIGURE 14–2 Minor surgical instruments (Courtesy of the Miltex Instruments Co., Lake Success, NY).

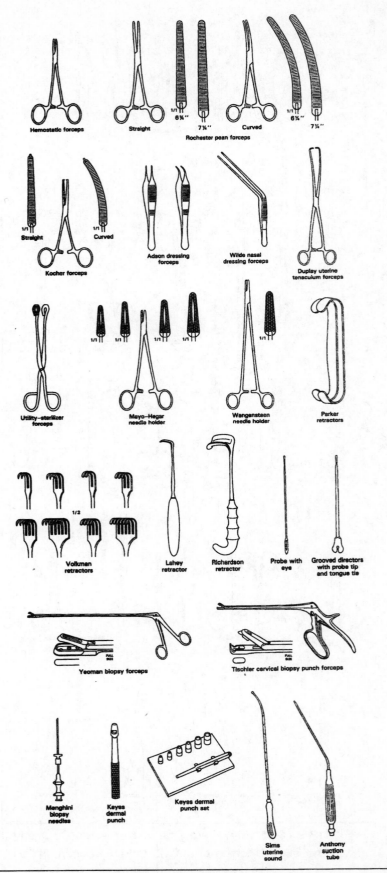

FIGURE 14–2 continued.

1. **Scissors:** for cutting (may be sharp/sharp, sharp/blunt, blunt/blunt)
   a. **Iris scissors:** small and sharp for precise cutting
   b. Straight or curved
   c. **Operative scissors:** to cut tissue during surgery
   d. **Suture scissors:** curved end helps get under sutures to cut them
2. **Forceps**
   a. **Splinter forceps:** to remove splinters
   b. **Allis tissue forceps:** grasping of delicate tissue
   c. **Sponge forceps:** tips wrapped in gauze for blotting and sponging
   d. **Mosquito forceps:** for clamping of very small vessels, and the like
   e. **Sterile transfer forceps:** for moving sterile items
   f. **Hemostatic forceps:** for clamping vessels
3. **Needle holders:** clamp needle in place for suturing
   a. Sutures
      • **Absorbable:** catgut
      • **Nonabsorbable:** silk, cotton, polyester, nylon, and stainless steel
      • Size 11-0 (thin) to 7 (thick)
4. **Biopsy punch:** punches out tissue for inspection under a microscope to see if it is normal
5. **Retractors:** pull back muscles or wound edges
6. **Scalpel:** sharp instrument for making incisions
7. **Cautery:** seals off bleeders and helps coagulate blood

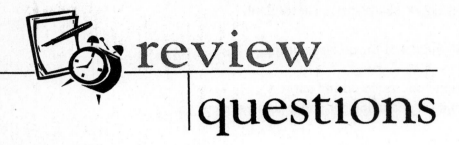

review questions

DIRECTIONS (Questions 1 through 10): Each of the numbered items or incomplete statements in this section is followed by answers or by completions of the statement. Select the ONE lettered answer or completion that is BEST in each case.

---

1. The single most important method of medical asepsis is
   A. handwashing
   B. dry heat
   C. ultrasonic cleaning
   D. sterilization

2. When you wash items with detergent and water, you have
   A. autoclaved them
   B. sanitized them
   C. disinfected them
   D. cold sterilized them

3. Complete destruction of all pathogenic microorganisms including spores is
   A. sterilization
   B. dry heating
   C. medical asepsis
   D. clean technique

4. To break the chain of transmission of many pathogenic organisms, you can provide
   A. a nonoxygen environment for anaerobic pathogens
   B. oxygen for aerobic pathogens
   C. moisture
   D. an environment of sunlight

5. The best defense against a needle stick is
   A. gloving
   B. gowning
   C. no recapping of used needles
   D. push needles in sharps containers

6. Round clusters of bacteria are identified as
   A. staphylococci
   B. streptococci
   C. spirilla
   D. bacilli

7. An instrument used to view the ear is the
   A. ophthalmoscope
   B. otoscope
   C. anoscope
   D. pinwheel

8. The surgical blade with the straightest, most pointed edge is a
   A. #10
   B. #11
   C. #20
   D. #22

9. Rules for maintaining a sterile field include which of the following?
   A. anything waist level and below is considered sterile

B. you may reach over a sterile field only once to straighten all items

C. items inside peel packs should be "popped onto" the sterile field

D. exam gloves should be donned prior to using items on the sterile field

10. An instrument used to clamp very small blood vessels is the

A. needle holder

B. sponge forceps

C. mosquito forceps

D. splinter forceps

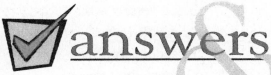
answers & rationales

1.

A. For medical asepsis, handwashing is the most important method of infection control. *(Fremgen, pp 354–55)*

2.

B. Sanitizing is washing with detergent or soap and water. *(Kinn, p 425)*

3.

A. Sterilizing is the only accepted method listed of completely destroying all pathogenic microorganisms including spores. *(Kinn, p 430)*

4.

D. Sunlight/ultraviolet rays work against the life of pathogens, therefore breaking the chain of transmission. Providing an environment that nourishes bacteria as answer a, b, and c do will not help break the chain. *(Fremgen, pp 345–46)*

5.

C. Making a rule never to recap needles is a good way to avoid needle sticks. Gloving and gowning help prevent contamination, but are no defense against needle sticks. You should never push needles into sharps containers. If they will not go in, the container probably is full. *(Fremgen, p 720)*

6.

A. Staphylococci are described as round, grapelike clusters. Streptococci are round chains. Spirilla are spiral shaped and bacilli are rod shaped. *(Fremgen, p 345)*

7.

B. An otoscope is for viewing the ear. Ophthalmoscopes are for viewing eyes, and anoscopes help view the rectal area. Pinwheels are for testing sensation. *(Fremgen, p 430)*

8.

B. The #11 blade is the sharpest, straightest of all the ones listed. *(Fremgen, p 485)*

9.

C. You should "pop" peel pack items onto a sterile field. Anything below waist level is considered contaminated. To reach over a sterile field makes it contaminated. Sterile gloves must be donned before working with items on a sterile field; exam gloves are not sterile. *(Fremgen, p 482)*

10.

C. Mosquito forceps

A needle holder grasps needles when suturing. A sponge forcep swabs areas or blots. A splinter forcep is used to remove splinters or briars. *(Lindh, pp 475–88)*

15

Clinical Equipment

contents

I. TYPES OF EQUIPMENT AND FUNCTIONS

A. *Thermometer:* **for reading body temperature**

    1. **Oral:** usually blue-tipped; has gradations of 0.2° F and ranges from approximately 94 to 106° F

        a. May be used under tongue or arm (reading will be 1° F lower than oral)

    2. **Rectal:** usually red-tipped with rounded bulb and same gradations as oral

        a. Inserted into rectal area (must be lubricated first) 1-½ inches for an adult, 1 inch for an infant (rectal temperature will be 1° F higher than oral)

    3. **Aural:** tympanic/ear thermometer resembles an otoscope; has disposable tips and is inserted into the ear for a few seconds until reading appears digitally (readings will be equivalent to oral)

    4. **Electronic thermometer:** usually has a disposable tip and can be used for oral, axillary, or rectal readings, which will be displayed digitally

B. *Sphygmomanometer (blood pressure cuff):* **for obtaining blood pressure**

    1. **Mercury:** has a vertical column of mercury for obtaining readings; gradations by 2 mmHg

    2. **Aneroid:** has a dial with a needle that points to numbers for readings; gradations by 2mmHg

C. *Stethoscope:* **for auscultation (listening) of heart, lungs, bowel sounds, and arteries during blood pressure checks**

D. *Physician's scales:* **for weighing patients**

E. *Microscope:* **for identifying pathogenic microorganisms, counting blood cells and platelets, and urinary casts and crystals**

F. *Autoclave:* **for sterilizing instruments by pressurized steam or gas**

G. *Ultrasonic cleaners:* **to clean and disinfect instruments using chemicals and sound waves to vibrate chemicals**

H. *Tape measure:* **to measure head circumference of babies, pelvises of pregnant women, and so on**

I. *Glucometer:* **to measure a patient's blood glucose**

J. *Autolet:* **a device used to prick fingers quickly and almost painlessly for capillary blood samples**

---

key concepts

• An excellent medical assistant is one who knows what equipment the physician will need before he/she asks for it. Know enough about all procedures to anticipate your physician's needs!

K. *Defibrillator:* gives electrical shocks to the heart to set it back in rhythm and stop fibrillation

L. *Audiometer:* machine for checking hearing; emits sounds of different levels for patient to identify

M. *Otoscope:* device for looking into the ear

N. *Snellen charts:* for checking distance visual acuity; Jaeger system for checking near visual acuity

O. *Ophthalmoscope:* instrument for looking into a dilated eye to see the retina

P. *Tonometer:* measures pressure in the eye to check for glaucoma (always use ophthalmic anesthetic drops prior to using a tonometer)

Q. *Ishihara vision book:* has numbers made of dots of one color against dots of another color background for patient to identify to check color vision

R. *Electrocardiography (EKG) machine:* checks heart for arrhythmias or irregularities

S. *Treadmill:* for stress testing a patient to see how much physical activity is appropriate and the heart's reaction to the stress

T. *Doppler:* instrument to magnify pulses and fetal heart sounds

U. *Spirometer:* measures lung capacity

V. *Sigmoidoscope:* scope that passes through the rectal area to the sigmoid colon to view the area for problems

W. *Wood's light:* purple fluorescent light used in dermatology to detect skin abnormalities

X. *Cast cutter:* cuts a cast to remove it from the patient's extremity; cast spreader: spreads the cast open after cutting it for removal

Y. *Cautery:* used to coagulate blood and to decrease capillary bleeding

Z. *Diathermy:* a form of heat to promote healing or reduce soreness of muscles

AA. *Centrifuge:* used to spin blood for hematocrits or urine for identification of casts and crystals; the formed elements will spin to the bottom and separate from the liquid portion

BB. *Hemoglobinometer:* determines the amount of hemoglobin in the blood

key concepts

• All clinical equipment has specific guidelines for maintenance. Always store manufacturer's instructions in the same room with the equipment. Keep spare parts available at all times!

CC. *Hemacytometer:* used in counting blood cells

DD. *Ear irrigation syringe/equipment:* used to irrigate cerumen (wax) or foreign bodies from the ear

EE. *Parrafin bath:* device used to melt and hold wax at a stable temperature. Patients can then dip hands or feet to coat and relieve joint stiffness.

FF. *Pulse oximeter:* measures saturation of oxygen in the blood.

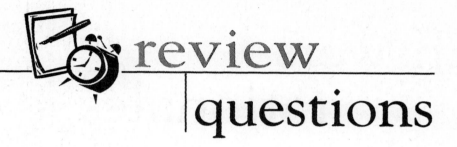

review questions

DIRECTIONS (Questions 1 through 10): Each of the numbered items or incomplete statements in this section is followed by answers or by completions of the statement. Select the ONE lettered answer or completion that is BEST in each case.

1. To check vital signs, you will use the following equipment.
   A. B/P cuff, otoscope, scales, thermometer
   B. scales, B/P cuff, stethoscope, watch, thermometer
   C. otoscope, ophthalmoscope, pulse oximeter, scales
   D. B/P cuff, stethoscope, watch, thermometer

2. The correct spelling for a B/P cuff is
   A. spygmomanometer
   B. sphygmomanometer
   C. sphygmonanometer
   D. spigmomanometer

3. The B/P cuff that has a dial rather than a vertical column is the
   A. aneroid type
   B. mercury type
   C. geratherm type
   D. aural type

4. A stethoscope may be used for
   A. auscultating bruits
   B. palpating pulses
   C. percussion of bowel sounds
   D. inspecting heart murmurs

5. A microscope may be used to
   A. read hematocrits
   B. grow pathogenic organisms
   C. identify urinary crystals
   D. count blood cells by photometry

6. A glucometer is used to
   A. record amount of glucose to be administered IV
   B. check blood sugar levels
   C. prick the finger
   D. check for eye disease due to increased pressure

7. The Snellen chart is used to check
   A. visual fields
   B. color vision
   C. visual acuity
   D. the retina of the eye

8. When an adult is in cardiac arrest, to get the heart restarted, you will need a/an
   A. diathermy machine
   B. lithotripsy machine
   C. defibrillator
   D. EKG (electrocardiograph)

9. To screen for glaucoma, you use the
   A. Ishihara method
   B. centrifuge
   C. tonometer
   D. PFT

10. You would most likely use a Wood's light in
    A. orthopedics
    B. dermatology
    C. gastroenterology
    D. bariatrics

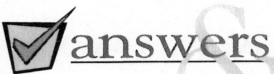

answers
& rationales

1.

D. Vital signs are pulse, temperature, respirations, and blood pressure.

To check pulse and respirations, you only need your watch to time them.

To check temperature, you need a thermometer. To check blood pressure, you need a stethoscope and a sphygmomanometer (blood pressure cuff). *(Fremgen, p 377)*

2.

B. *(Fremgen, chapter 20)*

3.

A. A dial is the aneroid type, while the mercury type is a column. Geratherm is a type of environmentally safe thermometer that works like mercury, and aural is an ear thermometer.

(Fremgen, chapter 20)

4.

A. Auscultating bruits means listening for abnormal sounds usually in the neck (carotid) artery. Palpating means feeling, percussing means tapping, and inspecting is looking in detail.

(Fremgen, chapter 20)

5.

C. In the listed answers, the microscope is only used when identifying urinary crystals. *(Lindh, p 896)*

6.

B. The glucometer is used to check blood glucose; the tonometer checks eye pressure in case of glaucoma; and a finger is pricked with a lancet or autolet. *(Kinn, p 932)*

7.

C. Visual acuity is checked when people try to read the Snellen charts. Color vision is checked with the Ishihara book. The retina is inspected by use of an ophthalmoscope after the eye is dilated. Visual fields are checked with various brand-named visual field machines. *(Lindh, p 689)*

8.

C. A defibrillator hopefully shocks the heart back into rhythm; a diathermy machine deep heats sore muscles; a lithotriptor crushes kidney stones. *(Fremgen, p 790)*

9.

C. A tonometer is a device to check eye pressure. A centrifuge spins at a certain speed to separate solid components from liquid, such as with tubes of urine or blood. A PFT is a pulmonary function test. *(Kinn, p 565)*

10.

B. Dermatologists use a Wood's light to luminesce diseases of the skin to help identify them. *(Kinn, p 704)*

16 Physician Assisting

contents

I. PATIENT PREPARATION

A. Vital signs: take and record all vital signs of each patient as a general rule

1. **Temperature:** may be done electronically by ear, mouth, rectum, or axilla or manually by mouth, rectum, or axilla.
   a. Digital readings or 0.2° F increments on nonelectronic thermometers
      • Average range is 97 to 99° F (36.1 to 37.2° C)
   b. **Normal reading:** 98.6° F (add 1° F under the arm, subtract 1° F in the rectal area)
   c. **Afebrile:** no fever
2. **Pulse:** usually taken at the radial artery (thumb side of the wrist area)
   a. Two to three fingers (but not the thumb) placed on the thumb side of the wrist
   b. Number of pulsations per minute counted (rate)
   c. Notation made as to whether or not rhythm is regular; notation is made as to volume type (weak, strong, bounding, thready)
   d. **Average range:** 60 to 100 beats/minute (varying with activity and body's physical condition)
   e. Types of arrhythmias of the heart (thus, an abnormal pulse)
      • **Bradycardia:** slow heartbeat (less than 60 beats/minute)
      • **Tachycardia:** fast heartbeat (more than 100 beats/minute)
      • **Fibrillation:** quivering of the heart's muscle resulting in inadequate pumping of the heart's blood
3. **Respirations:** after taking the pulse, one usually continues to hold the same position as for taking the pulse but looks at the patient's chest and counts breaths per minute
   a. One respiration equals one inhalation and one exhalation
   b. Shirt, back, or chest watched to notice breathing movements
   c. **Average range:** 12 to 25 breaths/minute
   d. Types of respirations
      • **Dyspnea:** difficulty breathing
      • **Bradypnea:** abnormally slow breathing
      • **Tachypnea:** abnormally fast breathing
      • **Kussmaul's:** showing air hunger when breathing
      • **Cheyne-Stokes:** no breathing (apnea) followed by gradually increasing breaths
      • **Hyperpnea:** increased rate and depth in breathing
      • **Hypopnea:** decreased rate and depth in breathing
4. **Blood pressure (BP):** sphygmomanometer and stethoscope needed; cuff goes around upper arm 1½ to 2 inches above the elbow bend with cuff centered over brachial artery; the stetho-

scope diaphragm is placed on the area of the brachial artery (not under the cuff)

   a. Blood pressure is the amount of pressure on the vessel walls as the heart pumps blood

   b. **Hypertension:** blood pressure readings consistently over 140/90

   c. **Hypotension:** if the patient is healthy, low BP is harmless

- **Orthostatic hypotension:** drop in BP due to sudden change from sitting to standing or from standing still for long periods
- **Shock:** a series of symptoms in which blood flow is inadequate for normal function; BP may be abnormally low or unobtainable

   d. Normal readings are below 140/90 with pulse pressure (difference between systolic, or top, reading, and diastolic, or bottom, reading) between 30 and 60

- Average pulse pressure = 40
- Abnormal pulse pressure = less than 30, more than 60

> ***key concepts***
>
> - For accuracy when taking blood pressure, always be sure the cuff is deflated completely before beginning.

B. Measurements (also called mensurations)

1. **Height:** can be checked by measuring rod attached to scales when patient stands on scales
2. **Weight:** place a paper towel on scales; assist patient to scales and move weights until scale is balanced
3. **Head circumference:** use tape measure to measure a baby's head
4. **Visual acuity:** may use Snellen chart to check patient's distance vision
5. **Spirometry:** used to check lung capacity
6. **Urinalysis:** measure urine for color and other components

C. *Chief complaint:* patient's reason for an office visit

1. Chief complaint must be known to prepare patient (e.g., if complaint is a sore throat, a strep test may be done and the patient asked to remove only clothing above the waist)
2. Duration of complaint (how long has it been going on?)
3. Medicines taken and whether they have helped
4. What makes it better or worse?
5. Other symptoms, together with chief complaint
6. Other pertinent data, such as past history, surgical history, family history, and social history

II. EXAMINATION TECHNIQUES

A. Draping and positioning

1. **Supine:** flat on the back with the legs straight

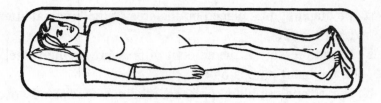

FIGURE 16–1A Horizontal recumbent position (supine).

   a. **Drape:** rectangular drape up to the chin
   b. Appropriate for examining any anterior area (on the front of the body)
2. **Dorsal recumbent:** flat on the back with the knees bent

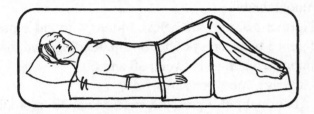

FIGURE 16–1B Dorsal recumbent position.

   a. **Drape:** rectangular or diamond-shaped with lower point of the drape between the knees
   b. Abdominal muscles are relaxed; therefore, position is good for an abdominal examination
   c. Rectal or vaginal areas can be examined
3. **Lithotomy:** flat on the back with the knees bent and in stirrups

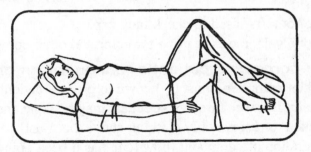

FIGURE 16–1C Lithotomy position.

   a. **Drape:** rectangular or diamond-shaped
     • **Diamond-shaped:** pointed flap may be lifted for examination
     • **Rectangular:** lower portion of the sheet is between the lower legs; it may be pushed upward with both of the assistant's hands and wrapped around the legs but out of the way of the examination area

   b. Appropriate for examination of female vaginal area, taking Pap smears, and so on

4. **Prone:** on the stomach with the head to the side

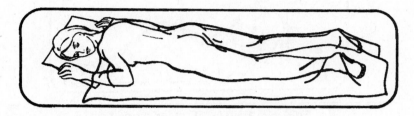

FIGURE 16–1D   Prone position.

   a. **Drape:** rectangular

   b. Appropriate for examination of the dorsal side of the body (backside)

5. **Right or left Sims:** on the right or left side with the lower leg slightly bent and the top leg sharply flexed

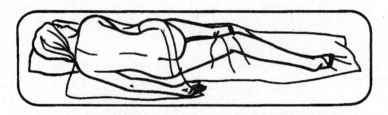

FIGURE 16–1E   Left Sims position.

   a. **Drape:** diamond-shaped drape with pointed end or flap over area to be examined, usually the rectal area

   b. **Left Sims:** position for taking rectal temperatures or giving enemas

6. **Trendelenburg:** on the back with the head lower than the feet

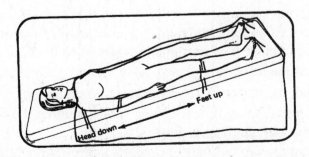

FIGURE 16–1F   Trendelenburg position.

   a. Rectangular drape

   b. Position for fainting (syncope) or shock recovery (unless head or chest injury)

key concepts

• Vital signs are called "vital" because they reflect the medical conditions of a patient that are vital to life.

key concepts

• Never think of vital signs as routine. You must be accurate, take them seriously, and report abnormalities for each patient.

7. **Fowler's:** sitting position

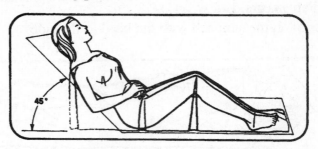

FIGURE 16–1G   Fowler's position.

   a. Patient is gowned, then a drape placed across the lap

   b. Appropriate for examining the throat, lungs, or any area above the waist; possibly the legs and reflexes

8. **Knee–chest:** on knees and chest with buttocks in the air

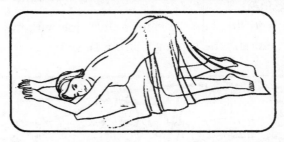

FIGURE 16–1H   Knee–chest position.

   a. **Drape:** diamond-shaped drape so that pointed end is at the feet and can be lifted for examination

   b. Appropriate for rectal examination, rigid sigmoidoscopy, and prolapsed uterus

B. Methods of examination

1. **Inspection:** generally looking the patient over

   a. Notations made of any deformities, unusual mannerisms, general health of the body, posture, and use of the extremities (arms and legs)

2. **Palpation:** examining by feeling specific areas of the body

   a. For example, breast examinations would be done by palpation

   b. **Bimanual:** using both hands, as in feeling the ovaries

   c. **Digital:** using one finger, as in rectal examinations

3. **Percussion:** tapping directly on an area or putting the fingers on an area and tapping the fingers

   a. **Use:** to discern outlines of organs to check for enlargement

   b. Appropriate for checking fluid-filled areas

   c. **Reflexes:** checked by percussion hammer or reflex hammer

4. **Auscultation:** listening to body sounds

   a. Lungs listened to symmetrically to compare one side to the other

key concepts

• If you are about to administer a medication or perform a treatment that may affect vital signs, always check and record them before and after the medicine or treatment is given.

    b. Auscultation of bowels may reveal a blockage or impaction

    c. Heart and pulse sounds may detect abnormalities in rhythm, for example

  5. Mensuration (measuring)

    a. Height and weight

    b. Head circumference of babies

    c. Chest circumference

    d. Pelvic measurements

    e. Length of extremities, angles of joints

    f. Fat measurements

  6. **Manipulation:** movement of an area, especially the joints

    a. Detection of the amount of movement in a joint or its range of motion

III. CLINICAL PROCEDURES

All procedures should be explained to the patient prior to performing them to alleviate the patient's anxiety. Hands should always be washed before and after each procedure. Universal precautions should always be followed using barriers (gloves, masks, etc.) appropriate to the procedure. Record all procedures in the patient's chart.

A. *Tine test:* screening test for tuberculosis

1. Inside of forearm is cleansed with antiseptic from inside out
2. Cap of tine test is removed and tines are pressed firmly while pulling the skin taut
3. Site of the test is recorded
4. Area observed after 48 to 72 hours and results recorded

B. *Scratch test:* allergy determination (tests may be invalid if the patient is taking antihistamine)

1. Site is cleansed (usually on the inside of the forearm or on the patient's back)
2. Identification of each area, leaving approximately 2 inches between sites
3. Each site is scratched with a separate sterile sharp instrument and a drop of allergen is added to the site
4. Observation of reaction (within 30 minutes) and results recorded
5. Site is cleansed

C. Patch test

1. Site is cleansed (usually on the inside forearm or on the patient's back)
2. Identification of each area, leaving approximately 2 inches between sites
3. Drop of allergen to each area with a cellophane adhesive patch covering or application of a gauze square impregnated with suspected allergen

4. Site is checked in 48 hours and results recorded

D. Pelvic exam
1. Patient in lithotomy position (in stirrups)
2. Vaginal speculum warmed with warm water or light warming tray unless sterility is needed
3. Doctor is given needed instruments (cytology brush, cervical spatula)
4. Microscopic slides for Pap test are smeared in correct area (V = vaginal, C = cervical, E = endocervical)
5. Fixative is sprayed on slides
6. Lubricant is transferred to the doctor's glove for a bimanual and rectal exam
7. Test for occult blood is prepared
8. Slides and the occult blood test are labeled

E. Visual acuity for distance
1. Vision of right eye (OD) tested first; therefore, the patient will put cover in front of the left eye so that the eye underneath the cover is open but not mashed
2. Indicate line on Snellen chart the patient is to read
3. Patient will stand back 20 feet and continue reading smaller lines until letters are missed
4. Record the smallest line read, indicating how many letters were missed (if the 20/30 line was read but the patient missed two, write 20/30-2)
5. Left eye (OS): same procedure

F. Irrigating eyes and ears
1. Outside area is washed (auricle/pinna for the ear, eyelids for the eye)
2. Patient holds the drainage basin and towel under the ear while flow is directed toward the upper ear canal or beside the eye so that the flow will be from the inner to outer canthus of the eye
3. Observe the area to be irrigated to identify material to be irrigated
4. Irrigate with a steady stream of liquid until all material is washed out
5. Ear/eye is wiped dry and procedure is recorded
   a. Ear of an adult is pulled upward and back
   b. Ear of a child is pulled down and back
   c. Eye is held open gently or upper and lower lids are rolled back with cotton-tipped applicators

G. Infant head circumference
1. Tape is placed around the head at an area right above ears and at eyebrows
2. Tape is pulled snug and measurement is recorded to nearest 0.01 cm

H. Bandaging and applying dressings

1. Protocol or orders are followed as to antiseptic application
2. Sterile dressing is applied to cover the wound adequately
3. Area is bandaged securely extending 1 to 2 inches above and below the dressing and taped as needed (may use tubular bandage for fingers, etc.)
4. Record is made of how the area looked, exact steps followed, and supplies used
5. Removal of old dressings and bandages: always cut through the bandage on the area opposite the wound site and record the amount and appearance of drainage
6. Tape is always pulled toward the wound when removing bandage

I. Removing staples and sutures

1. Area is cleansed
2. Staple remover is inserted under each staple and pressed together
3. Sutures: grasp each knot with forceps and cut the suture as close to the skin as possible to prevent drawing contaminated suture through the skin; suture should slip out easily
4. Staples or sutures should be counted to be sure all have been removed
5. Dress the area if necessary and record the procedure

J. Application of a hot or cold compress

1. Compress is never applied directly to the skin; there should be toweling between the compress and skin, or if the wound is open, use sterile compresses or towels
2. Temperature of the compress is checked before applying so as not to burn the patient
3. Compress is left for the prescribed amount of time, but the patient is consulted as to comfort

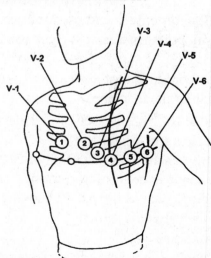

key concepts

• Be sure the electrodes of an EKG are well attached. If not, especially with a hairy chested male, it may cause the EKG stylus to burn out.

FIGURE 16–2 Precordial chest lead placement.

K. Performing an EKG

1. Preparation of the skin by rubbing the area briskly, applying gel, if needed, for better conduction, and attaching the electrodes to the following areas:
   a. Inside area of the right upper arm
   b. Inside area of the left upper arm
   c. Inside area of the right lower leg
   d. Inside area of the left lower leg
   e. Areas for chest or precordial leads
      - **V-1:** right of sternum at the fourth intercostal space
      - **V-2:** left of sternum at the fourth intercostal space
      - **V-3:** halfway between leads V2 and V4
      - **V-4:** midclavicular line at the fifth intercostal space
      - **V-5:** fifth intercostal space halfway between leads V4 and V6
      - **V-6:** horizontal to lead V5, but midaxillary under the left arm
2. Appropriate leads are attached to the electrodes
   a. Standard or bipolar leads
      - **Lead I:** electrical activity between the right arm and left arm
      - **Lead II:** electrical activity between the right arm and left leg
      - **Lead III:** electrical activity between the left arm and left leg
   b. Augmented or unipolar leads
      - **Lead AVR (augmented voltage, right arm):** electrical activity from the midpoint between the left arm and left leg, to the right arm
      - **Lead AVL (augmented voltage, left arm):** electrical activity from the midpoint between the right arm and left leg, to the left arm
      - **Lead AVF (augmented voltage, foot):** electrical activity from the midpoint between the right arm and left arm, to the left leg
   c. Chest or precordial leads (see leads V1-V6)
3. Standardization of the machine
4. Automatic mode for EKG is used or dials are set to each lead setting and each is run separately
5. Artifacts (interferences with recording of EKG) are corrected
6. Markings are made in areas of any unusual occurrences that change recording, such as the patient moving or coughing; re-record when the patient is settled
7. **Paper:** heat sensitive
   a. Smallest block: 1 mm x 1 mm; representing 0.02 second
   b. 300 blocks = 6-second strip

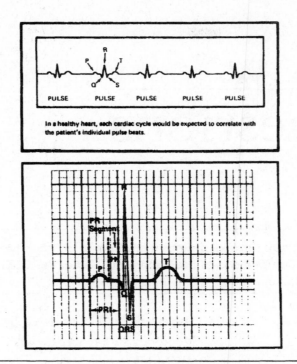

FIGURE 16–3 EKG recordings.

8. **Tracings:** P, QRS, T waves
   a. P wave: atrial contraction; indication that the SA node is working
   b. QRS: ventricular contraction
9. **Speed of tracing:** standard 25 mm/sec
   a. Can be slowed to 50 mm/sec if tracings too close to be read accurately

L. Body mechanics
1. Push, don't pull
2. Work area should be at or a little above waist level
3. Items should be carried as close to the body as possible
4. Stoop rather than bend
5. Stepping stool should be used rather than reaching
6. Correct patient transfer methods should be used

M. Catheterization
1. Urinary drainage of bladder
2. Method for obtaining sterile specimens
3. Irrigation or instillation of medicines into bladder
4. Procedure should be sterile
   a. Wipe each side of the labia or penis with indicated antiseptic, then wipe the middle
   b. Insert catheter until fluid drainage is observed
   c. Obtain specimen, or attach tubing to bag if indwelling

key concepts

PUBLIC HEALTH DUTIES:
The following must be reported:
• Births and deaths, certain communicable diseases, drug abuse, physical abuse, injuries caused by a violent act, criminal acts.

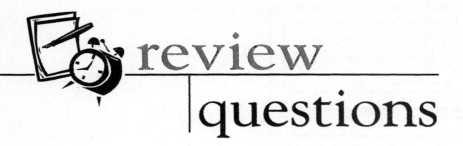

review questions

DIRECTIONS (Questions 1 through 10): Each of the numbered items or incomplete statements in this section is followed by answers or by completions of the statement. Select the ONE lettered answer or completion that is BEST in each case.

1. An average reading for normal blood pressure is
   A. 70/40
   B. 120/90
   C. 120/50
   D. 150/100

2. An average reading for normal oral temperature is
   A. 95.6 ° F
   B. 96.8 ° F
   C. 98.6 ° F
   D. 102 ° F

3. An average reading for normal respirations is
   A. 8 breaths/minute
   B. 12 breaths/second
   C. 16 breaths/minute
   D. 20 breaths/second

4. An average reading for normal resting pulse is
   A. 60 beats/second
   B. 70 beats/minute
   C. 80 beats/second
   D. 120 beats/minute

5. Hypertension is considered by most to be blood pressure readings over
   A. 140/90
   B. 130/90
   C. 130/80
   D. 140/80

6. A fast heartbeat more than 100 beats/minute is
   A. tachypnea
   B. bradypnea
   C. tachycardia
   D. hyperpnea

7. An examination position where the patient is on the stomach with the head turned to one side is
   A. supine
   B. prone
   C. Fowler's
   D. Trendelenburg

8. The most often used position for a Pap smear is the
   A. dorsal recumbent
   B. lithotomy
   C. left Sims
   D. knee-chest

9. The method of examination used by the doctor when performing head circumference is
   A. inspection
   B. palpation
   C. percussion
   D. mensuration

10. The scratch test would most often be performed in the
    A. obstetrician's office
    B. allergist's office
    C. ophthalmologist's office
    D. oncologist's office

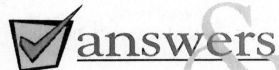
answers & rationales

1.

B. Average readings may vary, but 120/90 is normal average; 70/40 is low; 150/100 is high; and in c, 120/50, the pulse pressure is over 60. *(Fremgen, chapter 20)*

2.

C. Average normal temperature is 98.6° F. *(Fremgen, chapter 20)*

3.

C. 12–20 breaths per minute is normal average. 8 breaths/minute is slow and the other answers are in breaths per second. *(Fremgen, chapter 20)*

4.

B. Normal resting pulse averages 70. Below 60 is bradycardia (low); above 100 is tachycardia (fast). Pulse is stated in beats per minute, not per second. *(Fremgen, chapter 20)*

5.

A. Most refer to hypertension as over 140/90, but opinions are based on more than one reading and circumstances around the readings. *(Fremgen, chapter 20)*

6.

C. Tachycardia is more than 100 beats per minute. Bradycardia is less than 60 beats per minute. Tachypnea and hyperpnea are faster or deeper breaths than normal. *(Fremgen, chapter 20)*

7.

B. Prone is on the stomach; supine is on the back; Fowler's is sitting at a 45-degree angle with knees bent; Trendelenburg is head lower than feet. *(Lindh, p 457)*

8.

B. The lithotomy position when the female's feet are in stirrups is the position for Pap smears. *(Lindh, p 454)*

9.

D. Head circumference is measuring around a baby's head. Measurement is mensuration. *(Fremgen, p 410)*

10.

B. Scratch tests are performed to check patients' allergies. *(Kinn, pp 704–5)*

17 Laboratory Procedures

contents

I. LABORATORY TESTS

A. *Urinalysis:* collection and testing of urine

1. Physical examination of urine
   a. **Odor**
      - **Foul odor:** infection
      - **Fruity odor:** diabetes
      - **Ammonia odor:** urine that has been at room temperature for a while or has a high concentration of bacteria
   b. **Color:** normal is pale to dark yellow
      - **Red:** hematuria (urine with blood); some foods or drugs may cause redness
      - **Brownish:** bilirubin, bile, or melanin in the urine
   c. **Transparency:** clear is normal (newspaper can be read through it)
      - **Cloudy:** may have bacteria or excessive amounts of red blood cells, white blood cells, or other components; may become cloudy after standing at room temperature
   d. **Specific gravity:** ratio of the weight of a certain amount of urine as compared to the same amount of distilled water
2. Chemical examination of urine
   a. **Reagent strips:** dipped into the urine specimen and read by color changes in specified amounts of time
      - **pH (acidity or alkalinity):** below 7 = acid; above 7 = alkaline; 5.5 to 8 = average
      - **Protein:** negative to trace = normal
      - **Glucose:** negative = normal
      - **Ketones:** negative = normal
      - **Bilirubin:** negative = normal
      - **Blood:** negative = normal
      - **Urobilinogen:** 0.1 to 1.0 Ehrlich unit/dl = normal
   b. Confirmatory tests
      - **Protein:** treat urine with an acid to cause protein to precipitate; indicates protein in urine
      - **Sugars:** Clinitest tablet is the most common; tablet is dropped in urine and reacts if positive (Caution: may have false-positive results)
      - **Glucose tolerance test:** confirmatory for glucose
      - **Ketones:** Acetest tablet dropped in urine changes color if positive
      - **Bilirubin:** Icotest; color changes when tablet dropped on a urine-soaked pad if positive
3. **Urine sediment:** microscopic examination of urine (after centrifuging and pouring off the clear portion, called supernatant)

    a. **Red blood cells:** indicate trauma or disease (possibly contamination if patient is a female having menses); normal is 1 to 2 (use the high-power lens on the microscope)

    b. **White blood cells:** indicate infection; normal is less than 5 (use the high-power lens on the microscope)

    c. **Epithelial cells:** probably normal unless high number present from the kidneys; normal is 1 to 2 (use the low-power lens on the microscope)

    d. **Bacteria:** indicate infection and are abnormal (high power)

    e. **Yeasts or protozoa:** indicate disease and are abnormal (high power)

    f. **Hyaline casts:** usually normal (low power)

    g. Granular or cellular casts may indicate disease (low power)

    h. Amorphous urate, uric acid, and calcium oxalate crystals are normal in acid urine (high power)

    i. Amorphous phosphate, triple phosphate, and calcium carbonate crystals are normal in alkaline urine (high power)

    j. Cystine, tyrosine, leucine, cholesterol, and sulfonamide crystals are abnormal (high power)

  4. Drug screens

    a. Urine must be body temperature

    b. Specimen must be sealed in front of patient and signed by patient

B. Hematology

  1. **Hematocrit:** volume of red blood cells in a specific volume of blood

    a. **Low:** anemia or abnormal bleeding

    b. **High:** dehydration or polycythemia vera

    c. Performance of a microhematocrit test

      • Two heparinized capillary tubes of blood are collected

      • Tubes are placed in a centrifuge directly across from each other and with the sealed end against the gasket toward the outside edge of the centrifuge

      • Centrifuge is run with locked lid

      • Tubes are placed on a microhematocrit reader and averaged

      • Results are recorded

  2. **Hemoglobin:** oxygen-carrying component of red blood cells

    a. Hemoglobin is one-third of hematocrit

    b. **Hemoglobinometer:** use with capillary puncture to determine the amount of hemoglobin in blood

  3. **Erythrocyte sedimentation rate:** speed at which red blood cells settle

    a. Normal rate is slow: 1 mm every 5 minutes

    b. Abnormal rate is indicative of inflammation

key concepts

• Hemoglobin is one-third of hematocrit. Example: If hematocrit is 36, hemoglobin is approximately 12.

    c. Performance of a sedimentation rate test
- Venous blood is collected into a tube with an anticoagulant (a lavender-colored stopper is used)
- Tube is placed into a rack for 1 hour—with no movement
- Distance the erythrocytes have fallen is measured and recorded
- Amount of blood and tube size varies with method of testing

4. **Red cell count:** estimate of the number of circulating red blood cells
    a. Increase indicates erythrocytosis
- Polycythemia vera is an example
- People living at high altitudes may have increased cell counts

    b. Decrease indicates erythrocytopenia
- Usually, anemias are an example

    c. Manual red blood cell counting
- Red cells are mixed with a diluting fluid
- Hemacytometer (a glass slide made specifically with grids for counting blood cells) is filled
- Cells are counted; first row, left to right, second row, right to left, and so on, on side 1 of the hemacytometer
- Cells are counted only in four corner squares and center square of the large middle square of the hemacytometer
- Cells touching the lower or right edge of each square are not counted
- Findings are recorded; then side 2 of the hemacytometer is counted and recorded, the two sides averaged, and four zeros are added to the average

5. **White cell counting:** estimate of the number of circulating white blood cells
    a. Increase indicates leukocytosis
- Infections cause an increase
- Increase expected with leukemia

    b. Decrease indicates leukopenia
- Chemotherapy may cause a decrease
- Decrease expected with radiation

    c. Types of white blood cells
- **Neutrophils:** ingest bacteria (granulocyte)
- **Eosinophils:** aid during allergic reactions (granulocyte)
- **Basophils:** may absorb blood clots (granulocyte) (can remember all "phils" are granulocytes because they "phil" (feel) or look grainy under scope)
- **Monocytes:** aid in immunity and during infection (agranulocyte)
- **Lymphocytes:** B cells produce antibodies; T cells help immunity (agranulocyte)

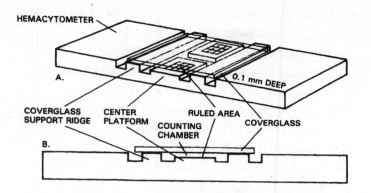

FIGURE 17–1 The hemacytometer.

d. Manual white cell counting
- Blood is mixed with white cell diluting fluid
- Hemacytometer is filled
- Cells within the four large corner squares are counted in the same manner and using the same boundary method as that used for RBCs
- Cells from slides 1 and 2 are counted and averaged, and multiplied by 50

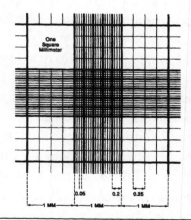

FIGURE 17–2 The hemacytometer has ruled areas for cell counting.

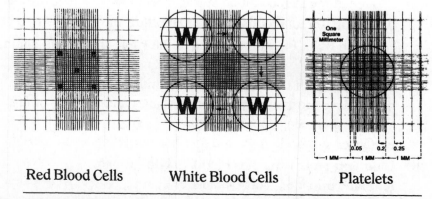

Red Blood Cells White Blood Cells Platelets

FIGURE 17–3 Areas for counting each type of blood cell.

6. **Platelet counting:** estimate of circulating platelets
   a. Increase indicates thrombocytosis
      • Increase appears after a splenectomy
      • Increase expected with polycythemia vera
   b. Decrease indicates thrombocytopenia
      • Chemotherapy may cause a decrease
      • Radiation may cause a decrease
   c. Manual platelet count
      • Blood and diluting fluid for platelets are mixed
      • Hemacytometer is filled
      • Platelets in the entire center are counted, using the same counting method and same boundary method as that used for RBC and WBC counting
      • Two sides are counted and averaged, then multiplied by 1000

7. **Blood smears:** for viewing blood components under microscope
   a. Small drop of blood is added to a clean slide near the end
   b. Another slide is used to pull back into the drop of blood until it spreads along the edges of the slide
   c. Second slide (that is in the drop of blood) is pushed forward to smear blood
   d. First slide is then dried, fixed, and stained

8. **Staining blood smears:** components of the blood may be seen better
   a. Slide is placed on staining rack with drainage system underneath
   b. Blood smear is flooded with Wright's stain and left standing
   c. Buffer is added and left standing
   d. Slide is rinsed gently and placed on end to dry
   e. Instructions are always followed for times (some quick stains can be dipped and rinsed in a very short time)

9. **Differential white blood cell (leukocyte) count:** finding percentages of each of the five types of white blood cells
   a. One drop of immersion oil is used; view under microscope the area of the stained blood smear where red cells barely touch
   b. Count 100 total cells using a pattern of moving down, then to the right, moving up, then to the right, then down again, and so on
   c. Record each type of leukocyte (white cell)
   d. Observe morphology (size and shape) and number of red cells and record observations
   e. Observe morphology and number of platelets and record

10. **Bleeding time:** evaluates blood's ability to clot
    a. Standard-sized incisions made
    b. Amount of time it takes to stop bleeding is timed and recorded

---

key concepts

ORDER OF DRAW
Evacuation Method
1. Blood cultures
   a. Aerobic
   b. Anaerobic
2. Red
3. Blue
4. Green
5. Purple
6. SST (gold, red, red/black)
7. Gray

11. **ABO slide typing:** determination of blood types
    a. Microscopic slide is marked as side A and side B
    b. Anti-A serum is dropped on the A side and anti-B serum on the B side
    c. Blood is dropped on each side and stirred with separate stirrers
    d. If agglutination (clumping) occurs on side labeled A, then blood type is A
    e. Agglutination on B side = blood type B
    f. Agglutination on both sides = blood type AB
    g. No agglutination on either side = blood type O

C. Bacteriology

1. Preparing a bacteriological smear
   a. Swab method
      - Swab of bacterial specimen is rolled onto a microscopic slide
      - Slide is air dried
      - Slide is passed through the flame of a bunsen burner
      - Slide is stained
   b. Culture tube or petri dish method
      - Inoculating loop is passed through the flame and a drop or two of water is added to the slide
      - Loop is reflamed
      - Loop is touched to bacteria, being careful not to touch the edges of the tube or petri dish, and bacteria is spread around in water on the slide
      - Slide is allowed to air dry, then is passed through the flame to heat fix

2. **Gram staining:** applying dye to bacteria for easier identification
   a. Slide is placed on staining rack with drainage system underneath
   b. Slide is flooded with crystal violet dye
   c. Slide is rinsed gently with water
   d. Slide is flooded with mordant (Gram's iodine), which causes the dye to adhere
   e. Slide is rinsed gently with water
   f. Decolorizer is added until clear (usually happens quickly)
   g. Slide is rinsed gently with water
   h. Slide is counterstained with safranin (red dye)
   i. Slide is rinsed gently with water
   j. Slide is blotted or air dried
   k. Oil immersion objective is used to view
   l. Purple = Gram positive
   m. Pinkish red = Gram negative

key concepts

ORDER OF DRAW
Syringe Method
1. Blood cultures
   a. Aerobic
   b. Anaerobic
2. Blue
3. Green
4. Purple
5. SST (gold, red, red/black)
6. Gray
7. Red

D. Occult blood (hidden blood in the stool)

1. Patient preparation and instructions for diet are necessary for accurate results and quality control
2. Specimen is obtained and smeared on the testing area
3. Reagent is added according to manufacturer's instructions
4. Positive or negative result is read and recorded

II. SPECIMEN COLLECTION

For all blood and body fluid collections, UNIVERSAL PRECAUTIONS MUST BE USED; hands are always washed before and after each procedure, gloves and other appropriate barriers are used, all hazardous waste is disposed of in a BIOHAZARD (red-labeled bag) container, and all sharps are disposed of in a puncture-proof container! Refrain from direct patient contact if you have open or exudative lesions.

A. *Urine:* first void in the morning is the most concentrated, and therefore is the best specimen for concentrated tests; refrigerate if not tested right away, or a fresh specimen may be obtained in office

1. **Midstream:** patient lets first few seconds of urination pass into toilet, then begins to urinate in specimen container
2. **Clean-catch:** used to determine if bacteria are present
   a. Area around the urethral opening is retracted
   b. Males wipe urethral opening three separate times using three separate towelettes
   c. Females wipe each side of urethral opening using separate towelettes, then front to back across urethral opening
   d. Urination begins, and midstream urine is collected

B. *Capillary puncture (finger, earlobe, or heel stick)*

1. Site is cleansed with alcohol and dried with sterile gauze or air dried
2. Skin is held taut and lanced quickly
3. First drop of blood is wiped away
4. Capillary tube (heparinized) is filled two-thirds full, holding it horizontally
5. Clean end of tube is placed in sealing clay
6. Pressure is applied to the puncture site to stop bleeding

C. *Venipuncture:* collection of blood from a vein (usually the median cephalic vein of the forearm)

1. Site is cleansed with alcohol using circular, inside-out method; let dry
2. Tourniquet is applied around mid-upper arm (not so tight that the pulse cannot be felt and for no more than 2 minutes)
3. Skin is held taut; needle (20 to 22 gauge) is inserted bevel up into the vein

4. Plunger is pulled back to aspirate blood, or if using Vacutainer method, tube is pushed up into Vacutainer holder unit but not punctured far enough to release vacuum until appropriately positioned in vein

5. Tourniquet is released before removing the needle

6. Needle is removed and pressure is applied to the site with a sterile gauze for several minutes

D. Collection tubes for blood

1. **Red:** no anticoagulant so serum will separate for testing purposes

2. **Purple:** EDTA (an anticoagulant) is used for hematology studies using unclotted blood (smears)

3. **Green:** for heparinized tests of unclotted blood other than smears

4. **Blue:** sodium citrate for coagulation tests

5. **Order of Draw**
   a. Evacuated Method
      • Blood Cultures-
        Aerobic Bottle
        Anaerobic Bottle
      • Red
      • Blue
      • Green
      • Purple
      • SST (gold, red, red/black)
      • Gray
   b. Syringe Method
      • Blood Cultures-
        Aerobic Bottle
        Anaerobic Bottle
      • Blue
      • Green
      • Purple
      • SST (gold, red, red/black)
      • Gray
      • Red

E. *Stool collection:* check feces for parasites or occult blood

1. Paper drape or cellophane wrap placed under toilet seat to catch stool, or the doctor may digitally examine patient and use stool sample from gloved finger

2. Wooden stick is used to obtain sample of stool to smear on testing area (if occult blood)

3. Wooden stick or gloved hands may be used to obtain sample for collection tube for other testing, such as for parasites

F. Throat swabbing
1. Patient is asked to open mouth and say "ah"
2. Tongue depressor is used to keep tongue out of the way while rolling sterile swab on both sides of the throat
3. Specimen is applied to culture medium or inserted into a culturette tube and labeled

G. Sputum collection
1. Best specimen is the first morning collection
2. Deep breath and productive cough are needed for deep lung secretions
3. Collection container should be sterile

III. NORMAL LABORATORY VALUES

A. Urine
1. Volume = 750–2000 ml/24 hours
2. Color = yellow
3. Transparency = clear
4. Specific gravity = 1.005–1.030 (stated as "ten o five to ten thirty")
5. Protein, glucose, ketones, bilirubin, blood, urobilinogen, bacteria, red blood cells are all negative
6. White blood cells = 0 to 4
7. Occasional epithelial cells
8. Occasional hyaline casts
9. Only cystine, leucine, tyrosine, and cholesterol crystals are reportably significant
10. pH = 4 to 8

B. Hematology
1. Red blood cells = 4,000,000 to 6,000,000 per mm^3
2. White blood cells = 4,000 to 11,000 per mm^3
3. Platelets = 150,000 to 400,000 per mm^3
4. Neutrophils = 50–60%
5. Eosinophils = 1–3%
6. Basophils = 0–1%
7. Monocytes = 3–8%
8. Lymphocytes = 25–40%
9. Hematocrit = 40–50%, males; 35–45%, females
10. Hemoglobin = 13–17 g/dl, males; 12–15 g/dl, females (*Note:* Hemoglobin is always one-third of hematocrit)
11. Bleeding time = 1–8 minutes
12. Sedimentation rate = 0–20 mm/hour (depending on the method used)
13. Occult blood or parasites = none should be found

14. Cholesterol = < 200 mg/dl (LDL = 60–180 mg/dl, HDL = 30–80 mg/dl)
15. Triglycerides = 40–150 mg/dl
16. Glucose = 70–115 mg/dl (fasting, serum)
17. BUN (blood urea nitrogen) = 9–25 mg/ml

IV. LABORATORY SAFETY

A. No eating or drinking in the laboratory

B. Laboratory jacket and closed-toed shoes are always worn

C. Universal Precautions are always followed

D. Work area is cleaned before and after each procedure (10% household bleach such as Clorox solution often used because it kills the AIDS virus on contact)

E. Hands are washed before and after each laboratory procedure

F. Safety glasses are worn as needed

G. Needle sticks or other incidents are reported promptly

H. Laboratories are equipped with safety devices such as a fire blanket, eye-rinsing station, fire extinguishers, safety glasses, and a body-wash station

I. Biohazard containers are provided for hazardous wastes; puncture-proof containers for sharps

J. All OSHA (Occupational Safety and Health Act) and CLIA (Clinical Laboratory Improvement Amendments) rules are followed

K. All MSDS (Material Safety Data Sheets) are read and filed

V. MICROSCOPE USE

A. *Three objectives* (magnifying lenses)
1. Low is magnified 10 times
2. High is magnified 40, 43, or 45 times
3. Oil immersion is magnified 95, 97, or 100 times

B. *Oculars:* 10x, 15x, and 20x

C. *Stage:* part on which slides are placed

D. *Condenser:* directs available light

E. *Diaphragm:* regulates amount of light

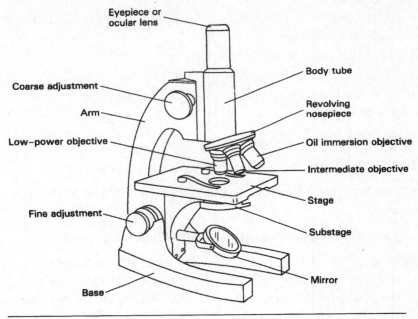

FIGURE 17–4 The microscope.

F. Adjustments for focus
1. **Coarse:** for low power only (after focusing with low power, other powers can be rotated into place; then use only the fine adjustment or slides will be broken)
2. **Fine:** used after object is initially found; clears image

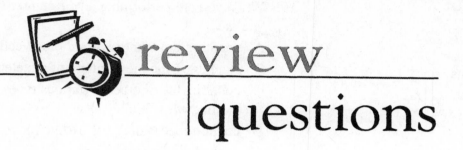

review questions

DIRECTIONS (Questions 1 through 10): Each of the numbered items or incomplete statements in this section is followed by answers or by completions of the statement. Select the ONE lettered answer or completion that is BEST in each case.

1. To check urine transparency, you might
   A. use a dipstick
   B. use a reagent
   C. put reading matter behind the container of urine and see how easy it is to read
   D. add a drop to a slide to examine under the microscope

2. Physical examination of urine includes
   A. protein
   B. pH
   C. color
   D. blood

3. An acetest checks for
   A. bilirubin
   B. sugar
   C. ketones
   D. protein

4. Urine sediment for microscopic inspection is usually obtained by
   A. drawing out and inspecting the supernatant
   B. straining the urine
   C. centrifuging and looking at the top portion of the urine in the tube
   D. centrifuging and looking at the bottom portion of the urine in the tube

5. An average normal reading for hematocrit is
   A. 12
   B. 20
   C. 38
   D. 60

6. Some rules to remember when performing an erythrocyte sedimentation rate are to
   A. take a reading after 3 hours
   B. periodically shake the rack the tube is in
   C. collect capillary blood for the sample
   D. collect blood in a tube containing an anticoagulant

7. Erythrocytopenia is indicated by
   A. an increase in red cell count
   B. an increase in platelet count
   C. a decrease in red cell count
   D. polycythemia vera

8. All the following are granulated WBCs except
   A. monocytes
   B. eosinophils
   C. basophils
   D. neutrophils

9. Chemotherapy may cause
   A. thrombocytosis
   B. leukocytosis
   C. decrease in infections
   D. increase in infections

10. When you are performing a "differential,"
    you are
    A. counting the number of red blood cells
    B. examining the morphology of platelets
    C. counting the number of various types of
       the five white blood cells
    D. counting red blood cells, white blood
       cells, and platelets

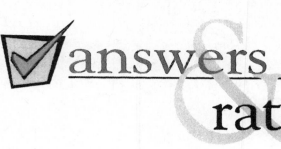

answers & rationales

1.

C. *(Kinn, p 855)*

2.

C. Color is the only answer in the physical examination of urine. The rest are in the chemical analysis. *(Lindh, p 887)*

3.

C. *(Fremgen, p 560)*

4.

D. To look at urine sediment, you have to centrifuge the urine to separate the solid portion from the liquid. The solid components will be at the bottom of the tube. You have to pipette the top liquid portion (the supernatant), before you can get a sample of the crystals and other solids. *(Lindh, p 894)*

5.

C. *(Lindh, p 895)*

6.

D. Blood must be collected in a tube with anticoagulant so it will not clot. The reading will be done in 1 hour. The tube must not be moved at all to obtain a proper reading. Venous blood is collected. *(Fremgen, pp 589–93)*

7.

C. Erythrocytes are red blood cells and -penia means a decrease. In polycythemia vera, there would be an increase in RBCs. *(Fremgen, p 599)*

8.

A. Monocytes are agranulocytes. The "phils" are granulocytes. Remember this by saying to yourself, "phils grainy" or "feels grainy." *(Tabers Cyclopedic Medical Dictionary)*

9.

D. Chemotherapy generally causes low blood counts. Therefore, very low platelets would mean less clotting and therefore, bruising, bleeding gums, and bleeding elsewhere. Low RBCs could mean low iron, anemia, and fatigue. Low WBCs may cause increased infections. *(Fremgen, p 595)*

10.

C. *(Lindh, p 949)*

18 Medication Administration

contents

I. COMMON DRUGS AND USE (ALWAYS CHECK PATIENT DRUG ALLERGIES BEFORE ADMINISTRATION OF ANY DRUG)

A. **Antihistamines**
1. **Claritin:** loratadine
   a. Use: rhinitis and seasonal allergies
   b. Caution with renal or liver disease
   c. Route: oral

B. **Spasmolytics/bronchial smooth muscle relaxers**
1. **Theophylline, Slo-Phyllin, Theo-Dur:** aminophylline
   a. Use: helps asthma and emphysema symptoms by relaxing bronchial spasms
   b. Adverse reactions: palpitations, tachycardia, and hypotension
   c. Route: oral
2. **Proventil, Ventolin:** albuterol
   a. Use: decreases bronchospasms and decreases asthma and emphysema symptoms
   b. Adverse reactions: tremor, palpitations, and tachycardia
   c. Route: oral or inhalation
3. **Adrenalin Chloride Solution:** epinephrine
   a. Use: decreases bronchospasms, decreases asthma and emphysema symptoms, is the drug of choice for severe allergic reactions (anaphylaxis), increases the heart rate and output, and increases blood pressure
   b. Adverse reactions: tremor, palpitations, and tachycardia
   c. Route: IM, SC, parenteral, or inhalation

C. **Antianginals**
1. **Inderal:** propranolol hydrochloride
   a. Use: decreases angina, arrhythmias, and hypertension
   b. Adeverse reactions: lethargy, bradycardia, and hypotension
   c. Route: oral
2. **Cardizem:** diltiazem hydrochloride
   a. Use: dilates coronary arteries, decreases angina, and is antihypertensive
   b. Adverse reactions: lethargy, arrhythmias, bradycardia, hypotension, and photosensitivity
   c. Route: oral
3. **Procardia:** nifedipine
   a. Use: dilates coronary arteries and decreases angina
   b. Adverse reactions: hypotension, palpitations, and dizziness
   c. Route: oral
4. **Nitrostat:** nitroglycerine (NTG)
   a. Use: increases blood flow in coronary arteries, decreases angina, and decreases hypertension

key concepts

• To find the 100 most prescribed drugs in the USA, obtain an April copy of the "Pharmacy Times" or search for "Pharmacy Times" on the Internet.

b. Adverse reactions: headache, weakness, orthostatic hypotension, tachycardia, and palpitations

c. Route: oral or skin patch (Transderm-Nitro: nitroglycerine transdermal system)

5. **Calan:** verapamil

a. Use: dilates coronary arteries, and decreases angina

b. Adverse reactions: dizziness, hypotension, and bradycardia

c. Route: oral

D. Antihypertensives/diuretics

1. **Tenormin:** atenolol

a. Use: decreases hypertension

b. Adverse reactions: lethargy, bradycardia, and hypotension

c. Tip: check pulse prior to administration; if less than 60, do not administer

d. Route: oral

2. **Capoten:** catopril

a. Use: decreases severe hypertension

b. Adverse reactions: leukocytopenia (decreased white cell count), tachycardia, and hypotension

c. Route: oral

3. **Lopressor:** metoprolol

a. Use: decreases hypertension

b. Adverse reactions: bradycardia, lethargy, and hypotension

c. Route: oral

4. **Maxzide, Dyazide:** triamterene hydrochlorothiazide (HCTZ)

a. Use: diuretic and decreases hypertension

b. Good choice when trying to avoid depletion of potassium (K+)

c. Route: oral

5. **Vasotec:** enalapril maleate

a. Use: diuretic and decreases hypertension

b. Adverse reactions: palpitations, arrhythmias, and hypotension

c. Route: oral

6. **Diuril:** chlorothiazide

a. Use: decreases edema and hypertension, and is a diuretic

b. Adverse reactions: hypokalemia (decreased potassium) and decreased blood cell counts (**Tip:** Encourage a potassium-rich diet)

c. Route: oral

7. **Lasix:** furosemide

a. Use: diuretic, for edema

b. Adverse reactions: agranulocytosis, orthostatic hypotension, and hypokalemia

c. Route: oral or IM

8. **Hytrin:** terazosin hydrochloride
   a. Use: diuretic, lowers blood pressure
   b. Avoid driving due to possible syncope
   c. Route: oral
9. **Prinivil:** lisinopril
   a. Use: lowers blood pressure
   b. Caution with impaired renal function
   c. Route: oral
10. **Norvasc:** amlodipine
    a. Use: lowers blood pressure
    b. Take vital signs to watch for hypotension
    c. Route: oral

E. **Cardiac glycosides**
1. **Lanoxin:** digoxin
   a. Use: strengthens heart contraction, used for CHF (congestive heart failure)
   b. Adverse reactions: weakness, lethargy, dizziness, hypotension, arrhythmias, and photophobia
   c. Route: oral
   d. Tip: check pulse before administration, if below 60, do not administer

F. **Antifungals**
1. **Monistat:** miconazole
   a. Use: vaginal candidiasis (fungal infection)
   b. Adverse reactions: burning, stinging, and irritation
   c. Route: topical (cream, lotion, or suppository), or aerosol
2. **Fulvicin:** griseofulvin ultramicrosize
   a. Use: ringworm and fungal infections
   b. Adverse reactions: headache, nausea, vomiting, and granulocytopenia
   c. Route: oral
3. **Mycostatin:** nystatin
   a. Use: infections caused by *Candida*
   b. Adverse reactions: nausea and vomiting
   c. Other forms: "swish and swallow" for oral thrush
   d. Route: oral, lozenge, or topical (vaginal cream)

G. **Anti-infectives**
1. Penicillins (patients often allergic)
   a. **Augmentin:** amoxicillin and potassium clavulanate
      • Use: urinary tract infections and upper respiratory infections
      • Adverse reactions: decreased blood cell count, nausea, vomiting, anaphylaxis, and superinfections due to overgrowth of nonsusceptible organisms
      • Route: oral or chewable

b. **Amoxil:** amoxicillin
- Use: systemic infections and urinary tract infections
- Adverse reactions: decreased blood cell count, nausea, vomiting, anaphylaxis, and superinfections
- Route: oral or chewable

2. Cephalosporins
   a. **Ceclor:** cefaclor
   - Use: urinary tract infections, upper respiratory infections, otitis media
   - Adverse reactions: decreased blood cell count, nausea, vomiting, and superinfections
   - Route: oral

3. Fluoroquinolines
   a. **Cipro:** ciprofloxacin hydrochloride
   - Use: urinary tract infections and upper respiratory infections
   - Adverse reactions: decreased blood cell count and superinfections
   - Route: oral or ophthalmic solution

4. Mycin drugs
   a. **E-Mycin:** erythromycin base
   - Use: upper respiratory infections, urinary tract infections, and prophylaxis for dental procedures
   - Adverse reactions: nausea, vomiting, hearing loss, superinfections, and anaphylaxis
   - Route: oral, topical, or ophthalmic ointment
   - May be drug of choice if patient is allergic to penicillin
   b. **Zythromax:** azithromycin
   - Use: mild to moderate infections
   - Do not take with food
   - Easy to use dosepack (oral)
   c. **Biaxin:** clarithromycin
   - Use: bronchitis, otitis media, upper respiratory infection, urinary tract infection, sinusitis
   - Do not take if pregnant or renal impaired

5. Sulfonamides (patients often allergic)
   a. **Septra, Bactrim:** trimethoprim and sulfamethoxazole
   - Use: urinary tract infections, bronchitis, and otitis media
   - Adverse reactions: decreased blood cell count, nausea, vomiting, photosensitivity, anaphylaxis, and crystaluria
   - Route: oral

6. **Achromycin:** tetracycline
   a. Use: broad spectrum antimicrobial
   b. Adverse reactions: nausea, vomiting, diarrhea, photosensitivity, and discoloration of nails and teeth

    c. Warnings: not to be given to children below age 8 (or pregnant women) due to tooth discoloration; do not take with dairy products or antacids

    d. Route: oral, topical, IM, or ophthalmic

  7. **Keflex:** cephalexin

    a. Use: urinary tract infections, otitis media, upper respiratory infections, and other infections

    b. Be careful giving to those patients allergic to penicillin

    c. May cause superinfection

    d. Route: oral

H. Gastrointestinal drugs

  1. **Zantac:** ranitidine hydrochloride

    a. Use: decreases ulcers and decreases gastric acid secretions

    b. Adverse reactions: decreased blood cell count, headache, nausea, and constipation

    c. Route: oral, or IM

  2. **Carafate:** sucralfate

    a. Use: decreases ulcers

    b. Adverse reactions: nausea and constipation

    c. Route: oral

  3. **Tagamet:** cimetidine

    a. Use: decreases ulcers

    b. Adverse reactions: decreased blood cell count, headache, and diarrhea

    c. Route: oral or IM

  4. **Prilosec:** omeprazole

    a. Use: ulcers, reflux, and esophagitis

    b. Do not crush delayed-release capsules

I. Sedatives/hypnotics

  1. **Halcion:** triazolam

    a. Use: decreases insomnia

    b. Adverse reactions: headache, nausea, vomiting, and rebound insomnia

    c. Schedule IV drug

    d. Route: oral

  2. **Dalmane:** flurazepam hydrochloride

    a. Use: decreases insomnia

    b. Adverse reactions: decreased blood cell count, lethargy, and headache

    c. Schedule IV drug

    d. Route: oral

  3. **Noctec:** chloral hydrate

    a. Use: decreases insomnia

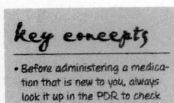

key concepts

• Before administering a medication that is new to you, always look it up in the PDR to check the dosage.

   b. Adverse reactions: decreased blood cell count, nausea, vomiting, and drowsiness
   c. Schedule IV drug
   d. Route: oral or suppository

J. Anti-inflammatory nonsteroidal drugs
1. **Feldene:** piroxicam
   a. Use: analgesic (decreases pain), decreases inflammation, and is antipyretic (reduces fever)
   b. Adverse reactions: increased bleeding, GI problems, photosensitivity, and anemia
   c. Route: oral
2. **Motrin, Advil:** ibuprofen
   a. Use: reduces inflammation, analgesic, antipyretic, and antiarthritic
   b. Adverse reactions: increased bleeding, and tinnitus
   c. Route: oral
3. **Naprosyn, Anaprox:** naproxen
   a. Use: antiarthritic, and analgesic
   b. Adverse reactions: increased bleeding and headache
   c. Route: oral
4. **Voltaren:** diclofenac sodium
   a. Use: antiarthritic, and after cataract surgery to decrease inflammation
   b. Adverse reactions: nausea, vomiting, stinging in the eyes, and increased eye pressure
   c. Route: oral or ophthalmic
5. **Relafen:** nabumetone
   a. Use: arthritis
   b. Risk of GI bleeding and ulceration
   c. Route: oral

K. Muscle relaxers
1. **Robaxin:** methocarbamol
   a. Use: decreases pain in acute musculoskeletal conditions
   b. Adverse reactions: headache, hypotension, nausea, GI problems, and anaphylaxis
   c. Route: oral or IM
2. **Flexeril:** cyclobenzaprine hydrochloride
   a. Use: decreases pain and decreases muscle spasms
   b. Adverse reactions: drowsiness, tachycardia, and dizziness
   c. Route: oral

L. Antianxiety agents
1. **Valium:** diazepam
   a. Use: decreases tension, muscle spasms, and seizures

key concepts

EIGHT RIGHTS OF GIVING MEDICINE:
• Right patient, Right drug, Right dose, Right route, Right time, Right documentation, Right technique, Right follow-up.

     b. Adverse reactions: lethargy, bradycardia, hypotension, and decreased respirations

     c. Schedule IV drug

     d. Route: oral or IM

  2. **Xanax:** alprazolam

     a. Use: decreases anxiety and tension

     b. Adverse reactions: drowsiness, hypotension, nausea, and vomiting

     c. Schedule IV drug

     d. Route: oral

M. Hormones/replacements

  1. **Premarin:** estrogen

     a. Use: abnormal uterine bleeding, prostate and breast cancer, and osteoporosis

     b. Adverse reactions: dizziness, increased risk of stroke or MI, nausea, vomiting, and weight changes

     c. Route: oral, IM, or vaginal cream

  2. **Lo-Ovral:** estrogen with progesterone

     a. Use: oral contraceptive

     b. Adverse reactions: headache, dizziness, thromboemboli, hypertension, nausea, and vomiting

     c. Route: oral

  3. **Triphasil:** estradiol and levonorgestrel

     a. Use: oral contraceptive

     b. Adverse reactions: headache, thromboemboli, and hypertension

     c. Route: oral

  4. **Provera:** medroxyprogesterone acetate

     a. Use: supresses ovulation, for abnormal bleeding, amenorrhea, and endometrial cancer

     b. Adverse reactions: dizziness, lethargy, nausea, and vomiting

     c. Route: oral or IM

  5. **Synthroid:** levothyroxine sodium

     a. Use: thyroid hormone replacement, stimulates metabolism, for cretinism, and myxedema

     b. Adverse reactions: nervousness, tremor, tachycardia, palpitations, and arrhythmias

     c. Route: oral or IM

  6. **Prempro:** conjugated estrogen and medroxyprogesterone

     a. Use: menopause; osteoporosis preventive

     b. Do not use with breast cancer or stroke patients

     c. Route: oral

  7. **Mephyton:** phytonadione (vitamin K)

     a. Use: increases prothrombin needed for clotting

    b. Adverse reactions: dizziness, hypotension, nausea, vomiting, anaphylaxis, and cardiac irregularities

    c. Route: oral, IM, or SC

  8. **Micro-K, Slow-K:** potassium chloride

    a. Use: replaces potassium

    b. Adverse reactions: hyperkalemia, hypotension, arrhythmias, confusion, nausea, and vomiting

    c. Route: oral

  9. **Feosol:** ferrous sulfate (category-hematinic)

    a. Use: iron replacement and anemia

    b. Adverse reactions: nausea, vomiting, constipation, and black stools

    c. Route: oral

 10. **K-Dur:** potassium chloride

    a. Use: potassium depletion

    b. Be careful giving to renal impaired patients

N. Antihyperlipidemic

  1. **Mevacor:** lovastatin

    a. Use: lowers cholesterol

    b. Adverse reactions: flatus, nausea, and lens changes in the eyes

    c. Route: oral

  2. **Lipitor:** atorvastatin

    a. Use: lowers cholesterol

    b. Caution with impaired liver function

    c. Route: oral

  3. **Pravacol:** pravastatin sodium

    a. Use: lowers cholesterol

    b. Caution with impaired liver function

    c. Route: oral

O. Antidiabetics/hypoglycemics

  1. **Micronase:** glyburide

    a. Use: increases insulin release, for Type II (non-insulin dependent) diabetes

    b. Adverse reactions: bone marrow aplasia, nausea, and hypoglycemia

    c. Route: oral

  2. **Glucophage:** metformin hydrochloride

    a. Use: blood glucose regulator

    b. May cause GI distress

P. Antiglaucoma ophthalmic drops

  1. **Timoptic:** timolol maleate

    a. Use: decreases pressure in the eyes

b. Adverse reactions: CHF (congestive heart failure), bradycardia, and headache

c. Route: oral or ophthalmic

Q. Antiacnes

1. **Retin-A:** tretinoin

   a. Use: decreases acne

   b. Adverse reactions: blistered skin and photosensitivity where used

   c. Route: topical only

R. Nonnarcotic analgesics

1. **Darvocet-N:** acetaminophen and propoxyphene napsylate

   a. Use: mild to moderate pain

   b. Adverse reaction: dizziness, headache, and euphoria

   c. Schedule IV drug

   d. Route: oral

2. **Ultram:** tramadol

   a. Use: moderate to severe pain

   b. Caution with respiratory distress or seizure patients

S. Anticoagulants

1. **Coumadin:** warfarin sodium

   a. Use: decreases vitamin K to decrease clotting; treatment for pulmonary emboli and MI

   b. Adverse reactions: hemorrhage, nausea, vomiting, alopecia, and decreased white blood cell count

   c. Route: oral or IM

T. Antidepressants

1. **Prozac:** fluoxetine hydrochloride

   a. Use: decreases depression

   b. Adverse reactions: headache, nervousness, nausea, and vomiting

   c. Route: oral

2. **Zoloft:** sertraline

   a. Use: depression and panic disorder

   b. Do not use with MAOI

   c. Route: oral

3. **Paxil:** paroxetine

   a. Use: depression and panic disorder

   b. Use with caution in patients with history of mania

   c. Route: oral

U. Anticonvulsants

1. **Dilantin:** phentoin sodium

   a. Use: controls seizures

   b. Do not stop taking abruptly; avoid alcohol

   c. Route: oral

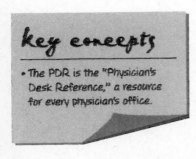

key concepts

• The PDR is the "Physician's Desk Reference," a resource for every physician's office.

V. *Immunizations:* **(American Academy of Pediatrics)**
www.aap.org/family/parents/immsch2000.pdf
1. **DTP** (diphtheria, tetanus, pertussis): give at 2, 4, 6, and 18 months, and at 4–6 years; tetanus and diphtheria every 10 years thereafter
2. **IPV** (polio): give at 2, 4, 6–18 months, and at 4–6 years
3. **MMR** [measles (i.e., rubeola), mumps, rubella (i.e., German measles)]: give at 12 months and 5 years
4. **Hib** (influenza): give at 2 and 4 months
5. **Varicella** (chickenpox): give after first birthday
6. **Hepatitis B:** begin series at any visit

Times and types of immunizations subject to change. Refer to American Academy of Pediatrics.

W. April *Pharmacy Times* **lists 100 most used drugs and categories each year.**

X. Controlled Drugs Schedules:
1. Schedule I: unaccepted medical use—very high abuse potential (LSD)
2. Schedule II: accepted medical use—highest abuse potential other than Schedule I (morphine)
3. Schedule III: moderate abuse potential (steroids)
4. Schedule IV: lower potential for abuse (Valium)
5. Schedule V: lowest potential for abuse (cough medicine with codeine)

II. ADMINISTRATION GUIDELINES

A. "Eight rights of giving medicine"
1. Right patient
   a. Identification of the patient without a doubt
2. Right drug
   a. Label is read three times
      • When removing medicine from the shelf
      • When pouring the medicine
      • When returning the medicine to the shelf prior to giving it to the patient
   b. Check the medicine against the doctor's order
   c. Verify the medicine when writing is not clear or spelling of the drug name is similar to another drug
   d. Ingredients may be the same but the names different
      • Generic: not sold under a specific trade name
      • Official: name is listed in the USP/NF (United States Pharmacopeia/National Formulary), the official list of standard drugs
      • Trade name: brand name given the same drug made by different companies

3. Right dose
   a. Check the package insert
   b. Use the PDR (Physician's Desk Reference) or other drug reference books to check dosage
   c. Check dosage measured against the dosage ordered
   d. Calculations of dosage
   • Knowledge of apothecary and metric system
   • General formula:

   $$\text{Dosage} = \frac{\text{Doctor's order}}{\text{Strength of medicine you have on hand}}$$

   Example: Doctor orders 250 mg; you have 50-mg tablets.

   $$\frac{250 \text{ mg}}{50 \text{ mg/tablet}} = 5 \text{ tablets}$$

   • Children's dosage:

   $$\text{dosage} = \text{patient age} \times \frac{\text{Usual adult dose}}{150 \text{ months (adult age)}}$$

   Example: $10 \text{ months} \times \dfrac{300 \text{ mg}}{150 \text{ months}} = 20 \text{ mg}$

   $$\text{Dosage} = \text{patient weight} \times \frac{\text{usual adult dose}}{150 \text{ pounds (adult weight)}}$$

   Example: $50 \text{ pounds} \times \dfrac{300 \text{ mg}}{150 \text{ pounds}} = 100 \text{ mg.}$

4. Right route
   a. **Oral:** (abbreviation—P.O.): by mouth
   • Safest but slowest route
   • Liquid, tablets, and capsules
   • Absorption is through the stomach and intestines (check if medicine should be taken on a full or empty stomach, with dairy products, etc.)
   • Timed-release capsules or enteric-coated tabs (do not crush)
   • If tablets are not scored, do not halve
   • Always shake suspensions
   b. **Buccal** (abbreviation—buc.): inside the cheek
   • Absorption is through mucous membranes (do not chew or swallow)
   c. **Topical** (directions will state how to apply)
   • Absorption is slow
   • Lotions are patted on; drops (gtt.) are for eyes or ears; sprays; bladder, wound, or vaginal irrigations
   d. **Rectal and vaginal** (p.r. or R. = rectal; p.v. = vaginal)

- Absorption is slow and irregular
- Cream, suppository, ointment (ung.), foam (ensure that patients receive instructions on how to administer so that they don't swallow suppositories)
- Rectal: for vomiting patient who can't keep medications down
- Effects: may be local

e. **Inhalation:** breathe in the medication
- Sprays, mist, steam, and puffs
- Use care in cleaning equipment

f. **Transdermal** (patch)
- Absorption is slow
- Systemic effects

g. **Sublingual** (under the tongue)
- Absorption is through mucous membranes
- Systemic effects
Example: Nitroglycerine tablets used in angina to dilate coronary arteries to increase oxygen to the heart muscle

h. **Parenteral** (injecting with needle and syringe)
- Absorption is rapid
- Intramuscular
- Intradermal
- Subcutaneous
- Intravenous (not done by medical assistants)

5. Right time
  a. Maximum effectiveness: drugs given at the correct time with the correct intervals of time between dosages

6. Right documentation
  a. Exact process of giving medication is written in the patient's chart

7. Right technique
  a. Technique is correct

8. Right follow-up
  a. Assess the patient for untoward reactions and allergies; note whether patient experienced pain decrease after taking pain medication; note changes in vital signs after medication administration, etc.
  b. Documentation in the patient's chart of follow-up
  Example: Vital signs taken; pulse 70 (after cardiac drugs)
  Example: Patient observed for 20 minutes with no signs of allergic or untoward reactions (after possibility of reaction to injection)

B. **Parenteral medication administration**
  1. Equipment

key concepts

CONTROLLED SUBSTANCE SCHEDULES:
- Schedule I: No accepted medical use; highest abuse potential
- Schedule II: High abuse potential
- Schedule III: Moderate abuse potential
- Schedule IV: Lower abuse potential
- Schedule V: Lowest abuse potential of all schedules

key concepts

SITES FOR INJECTIONS:
- Intradermal: lower arm, chest, back
- Subcutaneous: stomach, thigh, upper, outer arm, midriff
- Intramuscular: vastus lateralis, deltoid, ventrogluteal, and dorsogluteal (gluteus medius)

a. **Syringes:** must be sterile inside
   - Standard volume is 0 to 3 ml (cc)
   - Insulin is given in units (usual: 100 units)
   - Tuberculin or allergy syringes: for small dosages; calibrated in hundredths of a cubic centimeter
b. **Needles:** must be sterile and without burrs
   - Gauges: 18 to 21 for viscous medications; 22 to 26 for thinner, more liquid medications
   - Lengths: 3/8 to 5/8-inch for intradermal and subcutaneous; 1 to 1-1/2 inches for intramuscular
c. **Ampules of medication:** glass containers with bulb that will be broken or filed off
d. Vials of medication: containers with rubber stoppers (must be cleansed with alcohol prior to each use)

2. Intradermal injections
   a. **Sites:** into the upper layers of skin of the forearm or the back

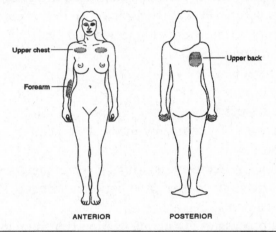

FIGURE 18–1 Intradermal injection sites.

   b. **Use:** allergy testing and TB testing
   c. **Amounts:** no more than 0.3 cc given
   d. **Needle size:** 3/8 to 5/8 inch; 26 to 27 gauge
   e. **Angle:** almost parallel to skin (10 to 15 degrees); will form a bleb when injected

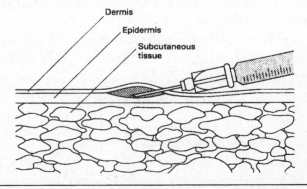

FIGURE 18–2 Intradermal injection.

   f. Tine tests pressed 1 to 2 mm in depth

   g. No aspiration needed prior to injection

3. Subcutaneous injections

   a. **Sites:** within fatty layers of skin on the upper arm, thigh, or abdomen

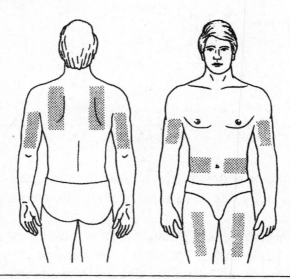

FIGURE 18–3 Subcutaneous injection sites.

> **key concepts**
>
> • The larger the number needle, the smaller it is.
> Example: A 28-gauge needle is smaller than an 18-gauge needle

   b. **Use:** insulin, local anesthesia, epinephrine, and heparin

   c. **Amounts:** 0.1 to 2 ml (cc)

   d. **Needle size:** 1/2 to 5/8-inch; 24 to 28 gauge

   e. **Angle:** 45 degrees (sometimes insulin is given at a 90-degree angle)

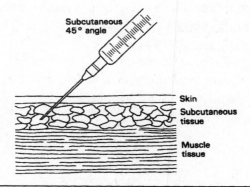

FIGURE 18–4 Subcutaneous injection.

   f. Aspiration is needed prior to injection (except insulin or heparin) to be sure injection is not intravenous

4. Intramuscular injections

   a. **Sites:** within a muscle

     • Deltoid muscle: upper arm, halfway between the top of the shoulder (acromion) and the armpit; the amount is 0 to 2 ml (cc)

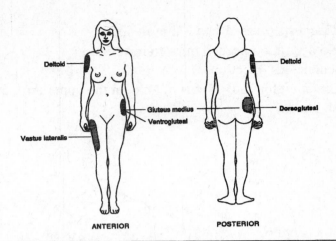

FIGURE 18–5   Intramuscular injection sites.

- Vastus lateralis muscle: midlateral thigh; the amount is 0 to 5 ml (cc); this is the safest parenteral route for infants and children
- Ventrogluteal site (gluteus medius muscle): on right side of the patient, place left palm of the hand on the greater trochanter and the index finger on the anterior, superior iliac spine. Spread the middle finger apart and inject into the "V" that is made by the index and middle fingers. The amount is 0 to 5 ml (cc).
- Dorsogluteal site (gluteus medius muscle): inject above an imaginary line from the posterior iliac spine to the greater trochanter of the femur; the amount is 0 to 5 ml (cc)

b. **Use:** penicillin and corticosteroid drugs

c. **Amounts:** 0 to 5 ml (cc); see individual sites for amounts

d. **Needle size:** 1 to 1 1/2-inches; 18 to 23 gauge

e. **Angle:** usually 90 degrees

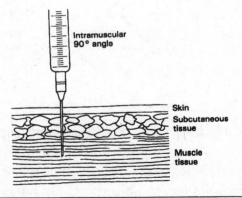

FIGURE 18–6   Intramuscular injection.

f. Aspiration is advised to be certain that needle is not in a vein or an artery

g. Avoid major nerves and vessels by location of correct injection site (especially avoid the sciatic nerve in the buttocks area)

5. Technique

a. Sterile technique is used: wipe area to be injected with a circular motion, inside out; use a sterile needle, sterile medication, and sterile area of syringe touching the medication (hands are always washed; Universal Precautions are always used)

b. Eight rights are used (right patient, right drug, right dose, right time, right route, right documentation, right technique, and right follow-up)

c. Medication is compared with doctor's orders and checked three times to ensure the correct drug is being used

d. Inspect the needle for burrs; inspect the medication for quality and expiration date

e. Wipe vial with antiseptic; air equal to the amount of medicine to be withdrawn is injected into the vial and the medicine withdrawn

f. **Ampule:** break and withdraw medicine (not necessary to inject air since no equalization of pressure is needed with an ampule)

g. Bubbles in a syringe are removed by gently tapping and pushing plunger to eliminate (recheck to be sure of correct dosage)

h. Needle is inserted quickly and at the correct angle: for subcutaneous injections, pinch up the skin; for intradermal and intramuscular, pull the skin area taut

i. **Aspiration:** to ensure a needle is not in a vein or an artery (no aspiration needed for intradermal; no aspiration needed for insulin or heparin injected subcutaneously)

j. Medication is injected slowly, the needle is removed quickly, and pressure is applied with sterile gauze at the site

k. Needle and syringe are deposited as a unit in a punctureproof container (no recapping is necessary to avoid possible needle stick)

l. Process is entered on the patient's chart, including documentation of eight rights.

Example: Patient: Jenny Hemby   12-12-01
2:15 pm 50 mg. Demerol IM right ventrogluteal area
for pain ordered per J. Langston, MD.
Tolerated well. Vital signs monitored before and after.
P-70, R-16, B/P-120/90. Patient states, "pain eased."

m. Observation of patient is necessary if there is a possibility of an allergic reaction or a change in vital signs

C. Prescriptions

1. **Date:** cannot be filled after a certain amount of time
2. **Patient data:** name and address
3. **Superscription:** Rx means "take"
4. **Inscription:** drug, dosage, and form
5. **Subscription:** amount to be dispensed
6. **Signature:** "Sig" means "write on label" the instructions to the patient (whether to take with food or on an empty stomach, how often to take, whether refrigeration is needed, etc.)
7. Refills: indicate whether or not to be refilled and how many times
8. Physician's signature: doctor must sign name and title
9. DEA number is usually imprinted on all prescriptions
10. Special DEA forms are needed for office prescriptions if controlled substances are to be administered in the doctor's office
11. Warning: keep prescription forms locked up
12. Verbal orders: be sure to record drug given and other pertinent information, but always get the doctor's signature showing that he/she ordered the drug. Check accuracy of the verbal order by repeating dosage and drug, etc., to the physician.

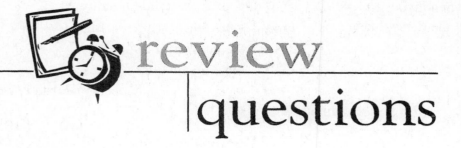

review questions

DIRECTIONS (Questions 1 through 10): Each of the numbered items or incomplete statements in this section is followed by answers or by completions of the statement. Select the ONE lettered answer or completion that is BEST in each case.

---

1. When using certain diuretics, you should watch for
   A. hypertension
   B. electrolyte imbalance
   C. increased energy levels
   D. potassium increases

2. Probably the most documented allergies are from
   A. sedatives and hormones
   B. antidepressants and antifungals
   C. sulfa and penicillin
   D. anti-ulcer drugs and antiglaucoma drops

3. Often, medicines are used for more than one purpose. The following results are often obtained by the same medication.
   A. antifungal/sedative
   B. gastrointestinal/antihypertensive
   C. diuretic/antihypertensive
   D. muscle relaxer/stimulant

4. Medication administration guidelines do not include
   A. right patient
   B. right drug
   C. right time
   D. right label

5. Rules for giving medicine do not include
   A. only cut tablets that are pre-scored
   B. always crush enteric-coated tablets
   C. shake suspensions before administration
   D. never swallow suppositories

6. Intradermal injection sites do not include the
   A. upper chest
   B. upper back
   C. buttocks
   D. forearm

7. The angle used for intramuscular injections is
   A. 15 degrees
   B. 30 degrees
   C. 45 degrees
   D. 90 degrees

8. The needle length for adult intramuscular injections is usually
   A. 1/2 inch
   B. 5/8 inch
   C. 1 inch
   D. 3 inches

9. A major nerve to avoid when giving an intramuscular injection at the dorsogluteal site is
   A. femoral
   B. abducens
   C. sciatic
   D. sural

10. "Sig" on a prescription indicates
    A. where the doctor is to sign
    B. the number of refills
    C. label instructions
    D. where the patient's personal data is written

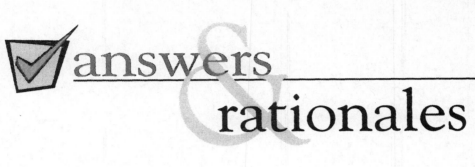
answers & rationales

1.

B. Certain diuretics sometimes cause electrolyte imbalances. When doctors prescribe these, they will often also prescribe potassium replacements due to the loss of potassium. *(PDR)*

2.

C. *(Kinn, p 1028)*

3.

C. Many times medicines that are diuretics also lower the blood pressure and vice versa. In item d, results of these medicines are usually opposite. *(PDR)*

4.

D. *(Kinn, p 1029)*

5.

B. Do not crush enteric-coated tablets. They are coated so they will be absorbed in the intestines and not in the stomach. This helps protect the stomach lining. *(Kinn, p 1005)*

6.

C. No injections are given in the buttocks; however, intramuscular injections can be given in the hip, in the dorsogluteal, or in ventrogluteal areas. Giving injections in the buttocks may cause you to hit the sciatic nerve or some major arteries. *(Fremgen, p 739)*

7.

D. A 90-degree angle is used for IM injections. A 15-degree angle is used in intradermal injections and 45–90 degree angles are used for subcutaneous injections depending upon circumstances. *(Kinn, p 1046)*

8.

C. You will use a 1 inch to 1-1/2 inch needle for adult IM injections. *(Fremgen, p 718)*

9.

C. You are avoiding the sciatic nerve when giving IM injections correctly. *(Fremgen, p 727)*

10.

C. *(Kinn, p 1000)*

CHAPTER

19

Emergencies and First Aid

contents

I. GUIDES FOR EMERGENCIES

A. *Scope of practice:* only administer treatment within limitations of profession and standard office protocol

B. *Listing of emergency numbers should be convenient:* 911 and poison control centers

C. Preventive measures should be practiced and taught to patients

D. Crash cart or tray should be on hand
1. Expiration dates should be checked regularly and documented
2. Inventory and restocking should be done after all emergencies
3. Drills should be practiced and roles assigned
4. Batteries should be checked and replaced as needed in battery-operated equipment; keep spares on hand

E. Emergency exits should be marked appropriately, fire extinguishers updated, and other emergency supplies and equipment marked and updated as needed; office staff must be aware of emergency procedures, locations, and equipment

II. CARDIOPULMONARY RESUSCITATION (CPR)

Always check for your own safety by inspecting the scene for hazards; use a mask or barrier between you and the victim.

A. *Responsiveness of patient:* ask, "Are you OK?"

B. ABCs of CPR
1. **A = Airway:** Is the airway open? Can the head be repositioned to open the airway? Avoid moving the head, however, if a neck injury is possible.
2. **B = Breathing**
   a. Look: Is the chest moving up and down?
   b. Listen: With ear over patient's mouth, do you hear breathing?
   c. Feel: With ear over patient's mouth and hand on chest, do you feel air or chest movement?
3. **C = Circulation:** When you feel the patient's carotid artery (beside the Adam's apple), is there a pulse?

C. *No breathing, but has pulse:* rescue breaths are needed
1. **Adult:** one breath every 5 seconds
2. **Child:** one breath every 3 seconds
3. **Infant:** one breath every 3 seconds

D. *No breathing, no pulse:* must initiate CPR, breathing for the patient and performing chest compressions

1. **Breathing:** adult and child—hold the patient's nose and blow breaths into the mouth (if using a mask, it will fit over the mouth and nose). Infant—rescuer's mouth over infant's mouth and nose.
2. **Chest compressions**
   a. Site
      • **Adult and child:** two finger widths above sternal notch or ziphoid process
      • **Infant:** place index finger sideways between nipples over sternal area, place middle and ring fingers next to index finger, lift index finger, and other two fingers are in place
   b. **Adult:** use both hands, one over the other (with heel of hand on sternum, fingertips up)
   c. **Child (8 years old and below, but not an infant):** use heel of one hand
   d. **Infant:** use two fingers only
   e. **Count:** one-person CPR
      • **Adult:** 15 compressions per two breaths for 4 cycles; then reevaluate need for CPR, continuing if necessary (rated 80 to 100 times per minute)
      • **Child:** 5 compressions per one breath for 20 cycles; then reevaluate need for CPR, continuing if necessary (rated 100 times per minute)
      • **Infant:** 5 compressions per one puff of breath for 20 cycles, continuing CPR after reevaluation of no pulse or breaths (rated at least 100 times per minute); brachial pulse checked instead of carotid pulse
   f. Two-person CPR
      • **Adult:** breaths by one rescuer, compressions by the other; compressor calls for switch when tired
      • 5 compressions per one breath for 20 cycles, continuing CPR after reevaluation of no pulse or breaths (rate = 80 to 100 times per minute for compressions)
   g. With adults "phone first" to get EMS and defibrilator. With children, "phone fast" or call EMS after giving 1 minute of CPR.

III. TYPES OF EMERGENCIES AND TREATMENTS

A. *Choking:* use Heimlich maneuver

1. Adult and child
   a. **Coughing and speaking:** leave patient alone; patient may be able to recover without help
   b. **Universal sign:** clutching throat (shows need for help); from behind the patient, put arms around (like a bear hug), and with one hand covering balled-up fist, swiftly give upward thrust below the ribs and above the umbilicus

    c. Upward thrusts are continued until patient coughs out foreign matter or until the patient becomes unconscious

    d. **Unconscious patient:** straddle and continue upward thrusts up to five times between the umbilicus and toward the rib cage using hand-over-hand method with heel of hand

    e. **No change:** if nothing is coughed out, insert hooked finger in back of throat (finger sweep) and try to expel the object from an adult (for a child you must inspect the mouth and do finger sweep only if an object is seen). Try to give 2 breaths.

    f. Upward thrusts, finger sweeps, and breaths are continued until the object is out or help arrives

    g. CPR is initiated, if needed, after the object is expelled

  2. Infant

    a. Five back blows between shoulder blades with head of infant downward, then five chest compressions (same placement as CPR)

    b. Back blows and chest compressions are continued until object is expelled

    c. When unconscious, mouth is checked after back blows and compressions to see if the object can be finger-swept out of the mouth. Breaths are tried.

    d. CPR is initiated, if needed, after the object is expelled

B. *Heart attack* (MI—myocardial infarction)

  1. **Symptoms:** pressure, squeezing sensation in the chest behind the sternum; pain may radiate to neck or shoulder, the patient may be extremely anxious, sweating, pale, and may have mild indigestion-like sensation; the patient may deny symptoms

  2. Complete rest is needed; nitroglycerine is given (if patient has it), 911 is called, CPR is initiated if needed, and an EKG is usually done. Defibrillation may be necessary.

C. *Stroke* (CVA—cerebrovascular accident)

  1. **Symptoms:** confusion, slurred speech, dizziness, weakness or paralysis on one side of body, and unequal pupils

  2. Allow complete rest, maintain the airway, place on side if secretions are draining, and call 911

D. *Burns*

  1. **First degree:** first layer of skin has redness but no blistering

    a. Immerse in cool water or cover with a sterile wet compress

  2. **Second degree:** deeper burn than first degree with redness and blistering

    a. Immerse in cool water 1 to 2 hours and cover with a dry sterile dressing

  3. **Third degree:** deeper layers and may include muscle tissue; nerve endings may be destroyed

  a. Cover with thick sterile dressing; if clothing is burned into and adhering to the skin; do not try to remove
  b. Infection is a risk; may need antibiotics
  c. Dehydration is a risk; may need IV fluids
 4. **Chemical burns:** rinse copiously and cover with a sterile dressing (if burn agent is a powdered chemical, try to brush it off first)
 5. Debridement may be necessary as the area heals and dead tissue sloughs off

E. Bleeding

 1. Direct pressure with sterile compress
  a. Use additional pads if necessary, but do not replace the old pad with a new one because you will disturb the clotting process
 2. Elevate injured part (if possible)
 3. **Pressure points:** apply pressure on the pressure point between the bleeder and the heart if direct pressure or elevation does not help

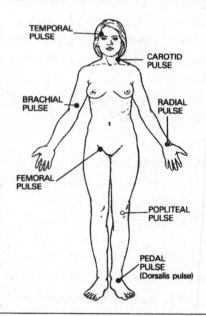

FIGURE 19–1   Pressure points of the body.

  a. **Common carotid:** above the clavicle, press backward
  b. **Temporal:** side of the face in front of the ear
  c. **Subclavian:** behind the clavicle toward the first rib
  d. **Axillary:** underarm area
  e. **Brachial:** above the bend of the elbow
  f. **Radial:** thumb side of the wrist
  g. **Abdominal:** press against the lumbar vertebrae toward the left
  h. **Femoral:** press against the groin area with leg abducted and rotated outward
  i. **Popliteal:** back of the knee

4. **Tourniquet:** use only as a last resort—always note the time tourniquet was applied (usually on patient's forehead), and use only as life or death measure

5. **Shock:** may occur with severe bleeding, internally or externally; monitor blood pressure

F. *Shock:* extremely low blood pressure

1. **Symptoms:** pale, clammy skin; weak, rapid pulse; low blood pressure; dyspnea; and weakness

2. **Treatment:** Use Trendelenburg position (legs elevated unless patient has a head or chest injury or dyspnea); maintain airway and continually check vital signs; keep NPO (nothing by mouth) and call 911

   a. **Traumatic shock:** fluids lost outside the cells, as in large burned areas

   b. **Hypovolemic or hemorrhagic shock:** internal or external blood loss; decrease in blood volume

   c. **Cardiogenic shock:** decrease of the heart's ability to pump

   d. **Septic shock:** severe bacterial infection

   e. **Neurogenic shock:** fainting, tone of vessels decreased and dilated; thus a drop in blood pressure and heart rate

   f. **Anaphylactic shock:** life-threatening allergic or sensitivity reaction to the extreme; edema, decreased blood pressure, dyspnea, and tachycardia

G. Poisoning

1. **Symptoms:** burns around the mouth, nausea, cramps, shallow breathing, loss of consciousness, and convulsions

2. Dilute poison by drinking liquids (water or milk)

3. Syrup of ipecac to induce vomiting unless contraindicated (as with corrosives and caustics); induce only if patient is conscious

4. Vomitus and container of poison should be carried to the hospital with patient

5. Activated charcoal is administered after vomiting to absorb residual poison

H. Convulsions

1. **Symptoms:** jerking, spasmodic movements of a part or of the entire body

2. **Treatment:** protect the head, maintain the airway, and nothing by mouth; after seizure, position on the side to promote drainage and prevent choking; call 911 if necessary

I. Fracture

1. Types

   a. **Simple:** no open wound

   b. **Compound:** open wound

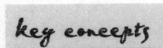

key concepts

• The newest research indicates that, with symptoms of a heart attack or stroke, it will help to take an aspirin.

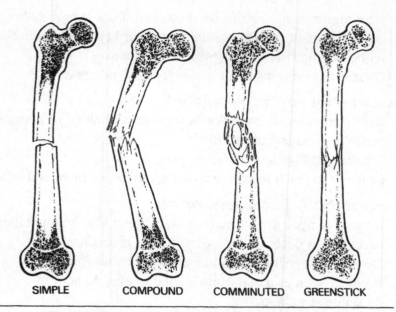

SIMPLE   COMPOUND   COMMINUTED   GREENSTICK

FIGURE 19–2 Different types of bone fractures.

key concepts

• Administer up to three nitro-glycerine tablets to patients whose doctor has prescribed it if they have signs of a heart attack.

    c. **Comminuted:** broken into more than two pieces

    d. **Greenstick:** part of the bone split away like a green stick

    e. **Transverse:** break across the bone

    f. **Oblique:** break slants across the bone

    g. **Spiral:** break spirals around the bone

    h. **Impacted:** part of the bone is compressed into another part

    i. **Depressed:** bone is driven inward

  2. **Treatment:** restraint to prevent movement, elevation (if possible), mild compression, splinting, and ice pack; x-ray is usually done and doctor may perform reduction of the fracture

J. Asthmatic attacks

  1. **Symptoms:** shortness of breath, choking, and wheezing

  2. **Treatment:** medicate with bronchodilators, inhalation therapy, and mucolytics

  3. Avoid excessive exercise, laughing, coughing, and stress

K. Insect stings

  1. **Symptoms:** edema, itching, pain, and anaphylaxis (shock-low blood pressure, dyspnea, and edema of the airways)

  2. **Treatment:** remove stinger without squeezing, apply ice, give antihistamines for itching and anaphylaxis, and give epinephrine if needed for full-blown anaphylactic shock

L. Diabetic coma/hyperglycemia

  1. **Symptoms:** dry, flushed skin; drowsiness, vomiting, air hunger, fruity breath smell, and intense thirst

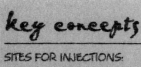

2. **Treatment:** increased insulin (however, if not sure if diabetic coma or insulin shock, best to give sugar because insulin shock without treatment can have dire consequences)
3. **Cause:** too little insulin, too much sugar, or stress

M. *Insulin shock/hypoglycemia*
1. **Symptoms:** moist, pale skin; excitement, shallow or normal respirations, and bounding pulse
2. **Treatment:** give food containing sugar
3. **Cause:** too much insulin, not enough to eat, or increased exercise

N. *Foreign body in the eye or ear*
1. Irrigate as necessary to remove the object; if instrumentation is necessary, a doctor should perform the procedure
2. Do not rub eye for it may cause corneal abrasions.
3. If object such as a nail is embedded in eye, do not remove, but do stabilize until arrival.

O. *Syncope* (fainting)
1. Loosen clothing and position the patient so that the head is below the heart

review
questions

DIRECTIONS (Questions 1 through 10): Each of the numbered items or incomplete statements in this section is followed by answers or by completions of the statement. Select the ONE lettered answer or completion that is BEST in each case.

---

1. When there is a pulse but no respirations in an adult, you
   A. begin CPR
   B. give two rescue breaths and wait for EMS
   C. give one breath every 5 seconds
   D. give one breath every 3 seconds

2. After establishing unresponsiveness of a patient, the very next step is to
   A. check pulse
   B. check breathing
   C. check for bleeding
   D. give two rescue breaths

3. After establishing that there is no pulse, your very next CPR step is to
   A. give two rescue breaths
   B. give compressions
   C. check for breathing
   D. check unresponsiveness

4. With an adult, the reason you call EMS prior to giving CPR is to
   A. gain access to a defibrillator
   B. get IV fluid access
   C. gain access to an EKG machine
   D. get trained personnel to do a tracheotomy

5. The Heimlich Maneuver is to be used on someone who
   A. has been poisoned
   B. is choking and coughing
   C. is drowning
   D. is choking and cyanotic

6. The correct hand placement when performing CPR on a child is
   A. two hands on the upper half of the sternum
   B. one hand on the lower half of the sternum
   C. two hands on the lower half of the sternum
   D. one hand on the upper half of the sternum

7. The ratio of compressions to breath for adult one person CPR is
   A. 15:2
   B. 5:1
   C. 15:1
   D. 5:2

8. The correct administration of compressions and breaths for an infant is
   A. 15:2 for 4 cycles
   B. 5:1 for 4 cycles
   C. 15:2 for 20 cycles
   D. 5:1 for 20 cycles

review questions

9. The ratio for CPR in a child aged 10 is
   A. 15:2
   B. 5:1
   C. 12:4
   D. 20:4

10. Sweating, chest pressure/pain radiating to the arm or shoulder may be signs of
   A. stroke
   B. heart attack
   C. choking
   D. migraine

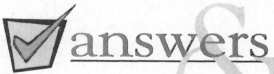

answers & rationales

1.

C. If there is a pulse, you do not give compressions, but if there is no breathing, you must give rescue breaths at the rate of one every 5 seconds for adults and one every 3 seconds for children and infants. *(American Heart Association)*

2.

B. After determining unresponsiveness, you follow the ABCs of CPR. Check A-airway, B- breathing, give two rescue breaths if no breathing, and C-circulation is checked by feeling for a pulse. *(American Heart Association)*

3.

B. When there is no pulse, your next step is to give compressions at the rate of 15 compressions to two breaths in one person adult CPR. All others have the rate of 5 compressions to one breath. *(American Heart Association)*

4.

A. Many adults will have cardiac arrest and will need a defibrillator to restart the heart. Without it, they may not be saved, so EMS needs to come quickly. *(American Heart Association)*

5.

D. Use the Heimlich when a person is choking and not speaking or coughing. They may be doing

the universal sign, which is putting their hands around their neck. When they are cyanotic, they need oxygen, so you must perform the Heimlich to try to get them to cough up the foreign body. *(American Heart Association)*

6.

B. On a child, you use only the heel of one hand on the lower half of the sternum. On adults, you will use the heel of one hand covered by the other hand. On infants, you will place one finger on the sternum between the nipples and lay down the next lower two fingers to perform compressions. *(American Heart Association)*

7.

A. *(American Heart Association)*

8.

D. 5:1 for 20 cycles *(American Heart Association)*

9.

A. A child aged 10 would be treated as an adult. Children aged 8 and below are given child CPR. *(American Heart Association)*

10.

B. *(American Heart Association)*

References

1. *Administering Medications* by Gauwitz, Glencoe, 4th ed., 2000.
2. *Appleton & Lange's Review for the Medical Assistant* by Palko, Appleton & Lange, 5th ed., 1997.
3. *Basic Laboratory Techniques* by Estridge, Delmar Publishing, 4th ed., 2000.
4. *Content Outline and Candidate's Guide;* free copy of guide obtained from AAMA Certification Department, 20 North Wacker Drive, Suite 1575, Chicago, IL 60606-2903. Phone 1-800-228-2262; FAX 1-312-899-1259.
5. *Delmar's Comprehensive Medical Assisting* by Lindh, Delmar Publishers, 1998.
6. *Essentials of Human Disease and Conditions* by Frazier, W. B. Saunders, 1996.
7. *Essentials of Medical Assisting* by Fremgen, Brady, Prentice-Hall, 1998.
8. *Lippincott's Textbook for Medical Assistants* by Hosley, Lippincott, 1997.
9. *Medical Law, Ethics and Bioethics in the Medical Office* by Lewis, F. A. Davis Co. 3rd ed., 1993.
10. *Medical Terminology: A Short Course* by Chabner, W. B. Saunders, 1991.
11. *Medical Transcription Guide Do's and Don'ts* by Fordney, W. B. Saunders, 2nd ed., 1999.
12. *Mosby's Medical Assisting Video Series,* Mosby, 1994.
13. *Program Review and Exam Preparation Medical Assistant* by Hurlbut, Appleton & Lange, 1st ed., 1998.
14. *Tabers Cyclopedic Medical Dictionary,* F. A. Davis, 17th ed., 1993.
15. *The Medical Assistant, Administrative and Clinical* by Kinn, W. B. Saunders, 8th ed., 1999.
16. *Understanding Human Behavior* by Milliken, Delmar, 6th ed., 1998.

Index

Page numbers in *italics* denote figures.

A

A-, 4, 8
AAMA. *See* American Association of Medical
    Assistants
AAMT (American Association of Medical
    Transcriptionists), 49
Ab-, 4, 7
Abbreviations, 15–16
ABCs of resuscitation, 208, 217
Abdominal quadrants, 17
Abdominal regions, 17
Abducens nerve, 34
Abduction, 27
ABO slide typing, 174
Abstracting journal articles, 126, 128
Accessory nerve, 35
Accounts payable, 123
Accounts receivable, 123–124
Accounts receivable ratio, 124
Acetaminophen and propoxyphene napsylate,
    194
Acetest, 181, 183
Acetest tablet, 170
Achilles tendon, 27
Achromycin, 189
Acne vulgaris, 23
   tretinoin for, 194
Acromegaly, 44
Ad-, 4, 7
Adding machine, 86
Address correction requested, 101
Addressing envelopes, 100, 101, 103, 104
Adduction, 27
Adeno-, 5, 9
Administration of medications, 195–201, 205.
    See also Medications
  abbreviations for, 15–16
  buccal, 196
  eight rights of giving medicine, 191,
    195–197, 203, 205
  inhalation, 197
  oral, 196
  parenteral, 197–201, *198–200,* 203–205, 214
  rectal, 197
  sublingual, 197
  topical, 196

  transdermal, 197
  vaginal, 197
Adoption, 116, 117
Adrenal gland, 42–44
Adrenalin Chloride Solution, 186
Adrenocorticotropic hormone, 42, 43
Advil, 191
Agent, 66
Aging of accounts, 129
Agranulocytes, 31, 183
AIDS support groups, 115
Airway management, 208
Albuterol, 186
Alcohol abuse services, 115
Aldosterone, 43, 44
-algia, 5, 10
Allergy
  anaphylactic shock, 62, 64, 212
  to anti-infectives, 188, 189
  skin tests for, 161–162, 167, 168
Allis tissue forceps, 145
Alphabetic filing, 92, 95, 97
Alprazolam, 192
Alveoli, 33
American Academy of Pediatrics, 195
American Association of Medical Assistants
    (AAMA), 49
  Code of Ethics, 49, 50
American Association of Medical
    Transcriptionists (AAMT), 49
American Cancer Society, 114
American Diabetes Association, 114, 115
American Heart Association, 114, 116, 117
American Lung Association, 115, 116, 117
American Red Cross, 114, 117
Aminophylline, 186
Amlodipine, 188
Amniocentesis, 41
Amoxicillin, 189
Amoxicillin and potassium clavulanate, 188
Amoxil, 189
Ampules of medication, 198
Analgesics, 191, 194
Anaphylactic shock, 62, 64, 212
Anaprox, 191
Anatomical position, 18, *18*
Anatomy and physiology, 21–46
Androgens, 43

Anemia, 32, 171
Angina pectoris, 32
  medications for, 186–187
Angio-, 6, 12
Angioplasty, 19, 20
Angry patients, 52, 54, 58, 59
Ankle bones, 24, 46
Anoscope, 141
Answering machines, 87
Anterior, 17
Anterior cruciate ligament, 26
Anti-, 4, 8
Anti-infective drugs, 188–190
Anti-inflammatory nonsteroidal drugs, 191
Antiacne drugs, 194
Antianginals, 186–187
Antianxiety agents, 191–192
Anticoagulants, 194
Anticonvulsants, 194
Antidepressants, 194
Antidiabetics, 193
Antidiuretic hormone, 42, 43
Antifungals, 188
Antiglaucoma ophthalmic drops, 193–194
Antihistamines, 186
Antihyperlipidemics, 193
Antihypertensives, 187–188
Anus, 28
Anxious patients, 59, 64
  antianxiety agents for, 191–192
Aorta, 31
Appendicitis, 45, 46
Appendix, 28
Appointments, 105–111
  canceled, 107, 109, 111
  categorizing of, 106
  determining time required for, 108, 110
  doctor delays and, 107
  establishing matrix for, 107, 108, 110
  guidelines for, 106–107
  patient information required for, 107, 108,
    110
  physician travel and, 121
  for referrals, 107, 109, 111
  scheduling of, 106
  triaging for, 109, 111
Arachnoid, 35
Arbitration, 66